I0448081

The AI Revolution in Healthcare

Transforming the Future

By
Dr Karuna Sharma

MBBS MRCGP DRCOG DFFP LOCMED

About the Author

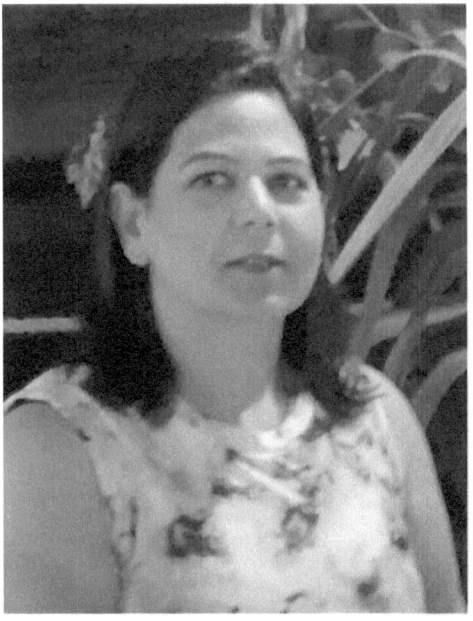

Hailing from Bihar in North Eastern India, Dr Karuna Sharma is a General Practitioner, teacher and trainer.

A graduate of Nalanda Medical College and Hospital, Dr Sharma currently resides in Farnborough, Hampshire, United Kingdom.

Fuelled by a passion and intrigue for the medical field and its future developments, Dr Sharma is also the author of "Medical Engineering, The Future of The Medical World".

Dedicated to my parents

Testimonials

A.I. is two words which is catching eyes of most around the world nowadays and seen as either a miracle that will solve all the problems at the drop of hat without any human error or a threat similar to dinosaur which will prove menace to its own creator devouring sources of his livelihood taking over most of his jobs rendering him jobless. Situation is not at all different in health sector too and among all technical advancements 'Artificial intelligence' is being taken with profound hope to remove all the fallacies and judgemental errors of doctors and paramedics and will do wonder by perfect predictions of outcome of patients' management. On the other hand, too much dependence on technology generates fear of more and more loss of clinical sense which we can already observe in most of upcoming young doctors developing disregard for proper clinical examination to explore and interpret investigation reports against physical findings.

(A)'Machine Learning' to learn from data, identify patterns and make decisions;(B) 'Natural Language Processing' to understand and interpret human language in order to transcribe doctors' prescriptions, analyse patients' feedback and detect potential adverse reactions from medical literature as well as (C) 'Deep Learning' to handle vast amount of datas and complex information using multi layer neural network capable of interpreting medical imaging and genomics data and predicting disease outbreaks, are three important subsets of AI used in health sector. Moreover AI robotics are of help assisting surgeons in performing intricate procedures with more precision and control particularly in minimal invasive surgeries reducing operating and recovery time with better outcome. AI will also be helpful in different administrative works including management of patients flow and triage. But putting at risk data privacy, securities, ethical and legal implications of machine made decisions as well as doctor- patient mutual trust are important hurdles AI will have to face. Explaining these intricacies in detail, author Mrs Karuna Sharma also reminds absence of empathy, emotions, compassion and nuanced humanitarian understanding in machines equipped with AI which play important roles in patient-care and emphasizes only supportive role for AI instead of considering as replacement option.

Inspired from grand success of her first book entitled 'Medical Engineering - The future of the medical world', she has come out with her second book 'The A.I. Revolution in Health Care - Transforming the Future' containing 12 Chapters covering every nook and corner of the subject in very balanced manner without any prejudice. Describing basic technical know how of Artificial intelligence in first chapter starting with overview followed by key technology and tools in detail, she dealt with current status of healthcare in chapter 2 enumerating current challenges and existing opportunities for improvement and then started looking for possible role of AI innovation in diagnosing diseases with predictve analysis for early detection in Chapter 3 alongwith personalised medicine and treatment plans with help of AI driven genomics in Chapter 4. After that she shifts her attention to Operational aspects of health care in Chapter 5 and beginning with analysis of its assistance in optimization of hospital management with proper resource allocation and streamlining administrative tasks, assessing compliance with regulatory standards as well as data analysis of performance metrics. Chapter 6 deals with how AI is going to help in enhancing patient engagement by working as virtual health assistant using chat bot and virtual consultation, wearable technology and remote monitoring, offering multi faceted approach to health care.

In Chapter 7 ethical and legal consideration about data privacy and security, decision making and accountability has been taken care of followed by discussion on its role in training and education of health personnels in Chapter 8 by integrating AI in medical curriculum with continuous learning and adaptation. Chapter 9 describes benefits of AI in tracking and managing epidemics like Corona and also use of population health analytics empowered by AI helping in revolutionizing public health management in areas of disease prevention, health promotion and policy making. Chapter 10 enumerates possible areas of its application in different clinical specialities like radiology, medicine, mental health, human reproduction and above all in surgical setup.

As author resides in UK and belongs to NHS, she also wishes if AI can transform NHS in Chapter 11 though she accepts that blending it with CQC's traditional practices would not be without challenges. Finally in Chapter 12 she ends up discussing thread-bare future of AI in global health care and concludes that confluence of AI and health care sector is going to be a revolution to redefine health care paradigm and patient care model on global scale holding a monumental promise and everyone will agree that future is both exciting and challenging whatever may be the outcome.

Finally I must congratulate Dr Karuna Sharma for possessing a prolific amalgamation of both engineering and medical brain. Only she with such wonderful devine gift could have written not only the present book but also her first one on medical engineering. She did justice by neither raising wild expectations about AI that may fall flat in future nor belittling its beneficiary potential in future upgradation of health sector on global scale. I will like to convey my best wishes for grand success of this quite useful book on current hot topic of AI.

Dr Sanjeew Kumar Chowdhary

MBBS MS (Surgery) PhD (Surgery) MCh (Plastic Surgery)

Surgeon, Author and Poet

Delhi, India

Sanjeew09@yahoo.in

26.07.2024

Testimonial for the Book, "The AI Revolution in Healthcare"

It is a pleasure to write this testimonial for the innovative book "The AI Revolution in Healthcare

Transforming the Future" written by Dr Karuna Sharma MBBS MRCGP DRCOG DFFP LOCMED.

Dr Sharma is an experienced General Practitioner in the NHS, an esteemed teacher and a brilliant trainer, fuelled with passion for transforming the future of health care through her knowledge in the field of Artificial Intelligence. Dr Sharma is also the author of the book "Medical Engineering, The Future of The Medical World", renowned for its significant impact on the medical technology field.

An important saying from Napoleon Hill states: "You are the master of your destiny. You can influence, direct and control your own environment. You can make your life what you want to be".As AI will have a big impact on our lives, this is the moment to influence, direct and control the AI revolution in a pragmatic way so that it transforms our future for the betterment of humankind. If someone is looking for the perfect guide on how to transform the future of healthcare with the rapidly developing AI revolution, I believe that Dr Sharma has done perfect justice to this topic. This brilliant virtuous investiture aims to help people through this transformative period and provides insights into the challenging journey ahead.

I wish her all the best and I am sure this book will be a great help to the doctors, medical students and all professionals who are passionately involved in this journey.

With best wishes,

Prof CK Sinha

Masters in Medical Ethics & Law (Special interest Artificial Intelligence and Medical Law), King's College, London.

FRCS (Paed Surgery, England), FRCS (Edinburgh), FRCS (Ireland), MCh (Paed Surgery), DA, MS, MBBS (Honours)

Consultant & Head of the Department,

Dept of Paediatric Surgery & Urology,

St George's University Hospital, London SW17 0QT

Author & Editor books entitled: "FUTURE DOCTORS", "Handbook of Paediatric Surgery" & "SARP series books"

28.07.2024

Testimonial for the Book, "The AI Revolution in Healthcare"

"The A.I in Healthcare" by Karuna Sharma takes you on a journey through the technological renaissance transforming modern medicine. Sharma paints a vivid picture of a future where algorithms and machine learning redefine healthcare, from wearables that predict illness to AI-driven diagnostics with unparalleled accuracy. This book is a thoughtful exploration of both the groundbreaking potential and the ethical challenges that come with integrating AI into healthcare. Sharma's balanced perspective makes this a must-read for anyone looking to understand the implications of AI on global health, offering insights that are as enlightening as they are essential.

Nick Ronald

Content marketer, Copywriter, Communications Coach & Public Speaker

Secret Influence Ltd ' 'Communicate & Persuade with Power'

Secret Influence TV

07957 211 196

10.08.2024

Testimonial for the Book, "The AI Revolution in Healthcare"

"Having worked with Karuna for 9 Years in the demanding environment of NHS primary care, it is useful for those of us in the latter part of our career to reflect on what has changed and how we work differently now and how that is going to change in the very near future.

Technology has brought us forward in huge strides in our daily medical lives and has enhanced patient care in many empowering ways, for example flash glucose monitoring in diabetes care, targeted biological and gene therapy in cancer treatments are interventions that we now wholeheartedly accept and expect... and struggle to fairly finance in a free-at-the-point-of-access medical system. By trying to improve people's health outcomes, we create health inequalities due to postcode lotteries. On a global scale this could be catastrophic making the most poor, poorer still.

Medicine is a mix of science and art. Talking to people, hearing stories and following a journey-building a narrative. Does this conflict with increasing use of AI- Where you take human interaction and intuition out of the equation? In a world where time, efficiency and data are king, is this what people want? Does this work for all scenarios? One would hope not. Then how do we decide who needs a computer algorithm to sort their problem and who needs a listening ear, real-world experience and human warmth? And as we approach the final generation of digitally excluded elderly, can a word of kindness be replaced by technology? It is a conundrum, as Karuna has wisely debated!!

Another question- Because we can do something, should we, would we? The impact of the digital footprint being eternal is a careful consideration that should not be forgotten. Data lives forever!

And as Karuna stated,"oh bureaucracy"! Never a truer word spoken especially in our UK NHS world. Whilst humans give the nod to the development and use of AI, does this take them away from their art of seeing, assessing and treating patients? Are we making ourselves redundant or are we enhancing our abilities? Building a legacy?

We hold people's lives in our hands-sometimes literally, mostly metaphorically. It is a big responsibility either way. Knowledge is power, power is knowledge. Use it carefully!"

A very well written book, I wish Dr Sharma all the very best!

Dr Nina Angela Durasamy

MBBS BSc MRCP MRCGP CIDC PGCert, Managing GP Partner

Fleet, Hampshire, UK

10.08.2024

Testimonial for the Book, "The AI Revolution in Healthcare"

"The AI Revolution in Healthcare" by Dr Karuna Sharma is an eye-opening exploration of how artificial intelligence is revolutionizing the medical field. This book provides a comprehensive overview of the ways AI is transforming patient care, diagnostics, and treatment.

From the outset, I was impressed by the depth of research and the clarity with which complex topics are explained. The author uses real-world examples to illustrate the profound impact AI is having on healthcare, making the content both engaging and accessible.

One of the most compelling aspects of The AI revolution in Healthcare is the focus on the ethical and legal considerations of integrating AI into medical practice. The balanced discussion of benefits and risks provides a nuanced perspective that is both informative and thought-provoking.

Overall, "AI in Healthcare" is an essential read for anyone interested in the future of medicine. It has broadened my understanding of how AI can enhance healthcare delivery and improve patient outcomes. I highly recommend this book to healthcare professionals, tech enthusiasts, and anyone curious about the intersection of technology and medicine.

Wishing Dr Sharma a huge success with this book.

Helen Grainger, Head of Nursing, Hart Health Partnership

Fleet, Hampshire, UK

15.08.2024

Testimonial for The Book- "The AI Revolution in Healthcare" by Dr Karuna Sharma

I have thoroughly read and enjoyed Dr Karuna Sharma's latest book entitled "The AI Revolution in Healthcare".

The book is an exceptionally well researched and written publication that addresses the current and potential future use and application of AI in the challenges facing Healthcare Professionals globally.

I particularly appreciated Dr Sharma's references to real-life examples that have already demonstrated the benefits of how valuable AI can be in the challenges presented by the practice and management of healthcare in today's society. The book addresses the multiple aspects of the use of AI in every possible area including the provision and management of medical facilities, medical education and research, medical diagnosis and treatment, surgical procedures, spread of disease and management of pandemics, and the use of pharmacological solutions. There is also reference to the wide use of AI to assist professionals with the challenges of demographics, language and the real need to share important information.

I fully recommend Dr Sharma's book as an essential read for anyone involved in or that has an interest in healthcare.

Grahame McCracken retired Managing Director and former owner of the Medical Molecular Imaging Company Bartec Technologies Limited.

Sandhurst, Berkshire, UK

20.08.2024

Testimonial for The Book- "The AI Revolution in Healthcare" by Dr Karuna Sharma

Artificial intelligence is fast becoming a part of everyday life, Dr Sharma's book offers insight into the use of artificial intelligence in healthcare. It explores how AI is currently being used in healthcare, the ethical considerations for its use and how it could help with the demand in healthcare systems.

Having worked in primary care for 14 years, and with a previous background in IT, I can see that AI will have huge benefits and a great impact in healthcare. There are many administrative and repetitive tasks that could be made quicker and easier, freeing up valuable resources for where it's needed most. With one prominent AI provider in primary care securing medical device status for its product, we are truly on the cusp of something revolutionising.

The AI Revolution in Healthcare explores the impact AI could have on transforming health outcomes around the world. An informative read from a highly experienced medical practitioner.

Steve Cardwell

Practice Business and former digital and IT support manager.

Fleet, Hampshire, UK

08.09.2024

Table of Contents

Introduction

Healthcare is on the cusp of a radical transformation, akin to a technological renaissance. Banish any notions of sterile waiting rooms and manual paperwork; we're venturing into the realm of algorithms, machine learning, and smart diagnostics. Imagine a world where your wearable device not only tracks your steps but also predicts your risk of developing a serious illness. Welcome to the future of healthcare.

It's easy to feel overwhelmed by the breakneck pace of technological advancements. Yet, it's crucial to harness this momentum for the betterment of public health. Artificial intelligence (AI) is not just another buzzword; it's swiftly becoming a cornerstone in healthcare innovation. From diagnosing diseases with unparalleled accuracy to personalising treatment plans, the potential applications of AI span a vast landscape.

The road ahead isn't devoid of challenges, of course. Ethical considerations, data privacy issues, and the need for robust training among healthcare professionals loom large. We have a responsibility to navigate these waters carefully, ensuring that this powerful technology serves humanity in the most ethical manner possible.

We'll delve into the current state of the healthcare sector, capturing both the exhilarating advancements and the stubborn hurdles that persist. Subsequent chapters will cast a spotlight on the myriad ways AI is being integrated into healthcare—from enhancing patient engagement with virtual health assistants, to transforming the operations of hospitals, and even tackling widespread public health challenges.

Our journey won't shy away from the ethical and legal labyrinths that accompany these exciting developments. We'll investigate what it means to make decisions when an algorithm is involved and scrutinise the implications for data security and patient privacy.

The integration of AI into global healthcare isn't a fleeting trend; it's a long-term pivot with implications that could redefine how we understand and manage health on a global scale. This book aims to guide you through this transformative period, providing insights and making sense of the changes ahead.

Chapter 1:
Understanding AI in Healthcare

The healthcare industry, often seen juggling the dual challenges of outsized patient demand and chronic staffing shortages, is now flirting with a new technological savior: artificial intelligence (AI). But before we get ahead of ourselves with grandiose visions of robot doctors and machine-driven miracles, it's pivotal to understand precisely what AI entails within this sector. In essence, AI in healthcare involves the application of complex algorithms and software to mimic human cognition in analysing medical data. This means everything from identifying patterns in diagnostic imaging faster than any human radiologist could, to predicting patient outcomes with a level of precision that's both awe-inspiring and a tad dystopian. Yet, despite all its shiny potential, AI remains both misunderstood and, to some, a somewhat unwelcome guest at the healthcare dinner table. So, as we embark on this journey, we'll endeavour to demystify the jargon, provide clarity on the technological underpinnings, and offer a candid discussion on the profound changes AI is heralding within the hallowed halls of medicine.

Overview of Artificial Intelligence

Artificial Intelligence (AI) is no longer the stuff of science fiction—it's here, making strides in various industries, including healthcare. This technology, often seen as the brain child of computer science and mathematics, is best understood as the ability of a machine to simulate human intelligence processes such as learning, reasoning, and self-correction. Going beyond mere automation, AI seeks to create systems capable of learning from experience and performing tasks that would typically require human intelligence.

At its core, AI involves the use of algorithms and complex data sets to create models capable of pattern recognition, decision making, and even prediction. It's not about replacing doctors but augmenting their capabilities to provide more accurate diagnoses, personalized treatments, and efficient care. The breadth of AI applications in healthcare is staggering, offering potential solutions to longstanding problems and inefficiencies.

One might wonder, what's driving this AI revolution in healthcare? The answer lies in the unprecedented access to vast troves of data generated by electronic health records (EHRs), mobile devices, wearables, and even social media. Data, as they say, is the new oil, and with AI, healthcare providers can extract valuable insights from this data mountain.

Now, let's talk about the types of AI making waves in healthcare. First off, we have *Machine Learning*, an AI subset that allows systems to learn from data, identify patterns, and make decisions with minimal human intervention. In hospitals, machine learning algorithms can analyse medical images for early detection of diseases like cancer, sometimes with greater accuracy than human doctors.

Another critical technology is *Natural Language Processing (NLP)*, which enables machines to understand and interpret human language. NLP applications in healthcare include transcribing doctors' notes, analysing patient feedback, and even detecting potential adverse drug reactions from medical literature.

Deep learning, a more advanced form of machine learning, uses multi-layered neural networks to handle vast amounts of data and complex patterns. It's behind some of the most powerful diagnostic tools, like those capable of interpreting medical images or genomics data. Deep learning models can predict disease outbreaks by analysing patterns in health records, travel data, and other relevant sources.

However, not all AI is created equal. A divergence exists between narrow AI, designed for specific tasks such as medical imaging, and general AI, which aims to perform any intellectual task a human can do. While narrow AI is already making significant contributions in healthcare, general AI remains largely theoretical at this stage.

A significant aspect of AI in healthcare is its role in predictive analytics. By sifting through historical patient data, AI algorithms can predict outcomes like disease progression and treatment responses, allowing for early intervention and tailored treatment plans. AI tools can also help identify high-risk patients who may benefit from more intensive monitoring, enabling proactive rather than reactive care.

Moreover, AI technologies like robotics are finding their place in the surgical theatre. Surgical robots, often AI-powered, assist surgeons in performing intricate procedures with greater precision and control. These technologies are particularly valuable in minimally invasive surgeries, reducing recovery times and improving patient outcomes.

Beyond the operating room, AI assists in streamlining administrative tasks, such as scheduling appointments and managing patient flow, which can significantly reduce the burden on healthcare staff. Intelligent systems can triage patients based on the urgency of their conditions, ensuring more efficient use of resources and shorter waiting times.

However, the integration of AI in healthcare is not without its challenges. Issues surrounding data privacy, security, and the ethical implications of machine decision-making loom large. There's also the matter of trust; both patients and healthcare providers need to trust these systems to make accurate and fair decisions. As AI becomes more prevalent, continuous ethical and legal scrutiny will be crucial to ensure it benefits all stakeholders equitably.

But let's not forget the human element. AI, despite its capabilities, lacks the empathy, compassion, and nuanced understanding that human healthcare providers bring to patient care. It's not about replacing healthcare professionals but empowering them with tools that enhance their capabilities. Training and educating healthcare professionals to work alongside AI will be vital in maximising the benefits of this technology.

From diagnosing diseases more accurately and quickly to personalising treatment plans, AI holds promise to transform healthcare, making it more efficient and effective. By leveraging the power of AI, we can hope for a future where healthcare is not only about treating diseases but also about preventing them, predicting them, and personalising treatments to the needs of individual patients.

In summary, the advent of AI in healthcare represents a significant leap towards redefining what's possible in medical science. As we stand on the brink of a new era, it's essential to navigate this transformation thoughtfully, considering the ethical, legal, and human factors at play. AI is not a magic bullet, but it's a powerful tool that, when used wisely, has the potential to revolutionise healthcare as we know it.

Key Technologies and Tools

Navigating through the labyrinth of **AI advancements in healthcare**, we encounter a trove of technologies and tools that promise to redefine how we diagnose, treat, and manage diseases. These advancements are not just futuristic concepts—they are actively being woven into the fabric of modern medical practices. Various forms of artificial intelligence have different applications, yet they all converge on one goal: enhancing patient outcomes and streamlining healthcare processes.

Machine learning (ML) is arguably one of the most prominent technologies in the healthcare domain. At its core, ML is about developing algorithms that allow computers to learn from and make predictions based on data. In healthcare, this can mean anything from predicting patient deterioration in a hospital setting to identifying potential disease outbreaks. What makes machine learning indispensable is its ability to process large datasets more efficiently than humans can, identifying patterns that might be invisible to human eyes.

Deep learning, a subset of machine learning, takes it a step further. Deep learning models use neural networks with many layers, enabling them to handle more complex tasks. For instance, these algorithms can analyse medical images like MRIs and X-rays, often outperforming human radiologists in accuracy and speed. Imagine a world where a machine can detect tumour cells in a fraction of the time it takes for a human to do so. That's no longer science fiction; it's current reality.

Natural Language Processing (NLP) is another pivotal technology. NLP allows computers to understand, interpret, and respond to human language in a valuable way. In healthcare, NLP can be used to sift through vast amounts of unstructured data, such as electronic health records (EHRs), to extract meaningful insights. This can significantly enhance clinical decision support systems, reduce the administrative burden on healthcare providers, and help in identifying trends and correlations that can lead to better patient care.

Virtual healthcare has risen from the shadows to the limelight, thanks to telehealth platforms and virtual consultations. Behind the scenes of these innovations is the quiet, yet monumental, work of AI-driven chatbots and virtual health assistants. They manage everything from scheduling appointments to offering preliminary diagnoses based on patient-reported symptoms. These tools are not just for convenience; they play a critical role in extending healthcare access to remote or underserved areas.

We mustn't overlook the importance of data security tools in this landscape. With the rise of AI, there is a parallel increase in the volume and sensitivity of data generated and stored. Healthcare providers are turning to advanced cybersecurity protocols to protect patient information. Blockchain technology, often associated with cryptocurrency, is gaining traction for its ability to offer secure data exchanges and ensure the integrity of medical records. Blockchain's decentralised nature means it can provide robust security mechanisms that are crucial for maintaining patient trust and regulatory compliance.

Wearable technology, embedded with sensors and connected to AI systems, is another game-changer. From smartwatches that monitor heart rates to more advanced devices that can track glucose levels in diabetics, wearables provide real-time data that can warn of impending medical issues. These devices feed data into AI algorithms, which then analyse it to provide actionable insights. It's like having a doctor on your wrist, constantly monitoring your vital signs and alerting you or your physician at the first sign of trouble.

Another critical tool in the AI healthcare toolkit is predictive analytics. Predictive analytics leverages historical data to forecast future events. In the context of healthcare, this could mean predicting a patient's risk of developing a chronic disease, such as diabetes or hypertension, based on existing health data. Early interventions can then be employed to prevent or mitigate these conditions, dramatically improving patient outcomes and reducing healthcare costs.

Robotic Process Automation (RPA) is yet another technology making waves. RPA involves using software robots to automate repetitive, rule-based tasks. In healthcare, this can be as mundane as managing patient records or as intricate as ensuring compliance with regulatory requirements. By freeing up human resources from these tasks, RPA allows healthcare professionals to focus more on patient-centred activities.

We're also seeing a surge in the application of AI in genomics. The ability to analyse genetic data quickly and accurately can lead to breakthroughs in personalised medicine. AI algorithms can identify genetic markers for diseases, paving the way for treatments tailored to the individual's genetic makeup. This level of precision wasn't possible before, and it holds promise for treating illnesses that have so far eluded conventional medicine.

Imagine a scenario where clinical trials are not sample-based but individualised to the genetic profile of each participant. AI-driven platforms can expedite this process by identifying suitable candidates, monitoring ongoing trials in real-time, and analysing results more rapidly and accurately. This could lead to faster drug development cycles compared to the traditional methods that often take years, if not decades.

Supply chain management in healthcare also benefits from AI technologies. AI can optimise the supply chain for pharmaceuticals and medical equipment by predicting demand based on historical data and trends. This ensures that healthcare facilities are adequately stocked without overspending on surplus inventory. It's a balancing act that AI handles remarkably well, saving time and resources that can be redirected to more critical areas.

Let's not forget about AI's role in streamlining healthcare operations. Advanced scheduling systems powered by AI can manage appointment bookings more efficiently, reducing wait times and no-show rates. AI can also assist in staff allocation, ensuring that the right number of healthcare providers are available at peak times, thereby optimising the utilisation of human resources.

In emergency care, AI tools can be lifesaving. Predictive analytics can forecast patient load in emergency departments, helping hospitals prepare in advance for sudden surges in patient numbers. Wearable devices and mobile apps connected to AI alert systems can notify healthcare providers about critical health events in real-time, enabling faster and more accurate response times.

While the current technologies are impressive, the pipeline of potential tools is equally exciting. Quantum computing, for example, holds the promise of solving complex medical problems at speeds inconceivable with current technology. Though still in its nascent stages, quantum computing could revolutionise the field of drug discovery and genomics, among other areas.

In summary, the arsenal of AI technologies and tools at our disposal today is nothing short of revolutionary. From machine learning and deep learning to natural language processing, wearable tech, and blockchain, each of these innovations plays a pivotal role in transforming healthcare. These tools are changing how we diagnose, treat, and manage health conditions, ultimately enhancing patient care and operational efficiency. It's an exciting time for healthcare, and the future holds even greater promise.

Chapter 2:
The Current State of Healthcare

A t this very moment, the healthcare sector is caught in a complex dance of advances and setbacks. We're seeing technological marvels emerge, promising to revolutionise patient care, while simultaneously grappling with age-old challenges, such as resource scarcity and bureaucratic red tape. The cracks in the system are more pronounced than ever, as healthcare providers struggle with everything from outdated electronic health records to overwhelming patient loads. Yet, these very pain points are also opportunities in disguise. With the right investments in technology and innovation, there's potential to metamorphose the landscape — reducing inefficiencies, improving patient outcomes, and ultimately, delivering a more equitable healthcare experience. It's a predicament wrapped in progress, and the status quo is anything but static.

Existing Challenges

The healthcare sector is undoubtedly one of the pillars of modern society, yet it's riddled with problems that would make even the most stoic patients clutch their hospital gowns in frustration. Let's start with the most glaring issue—access to care. Public healthcare systems in many countries, especially the UK, are groaning under the weight of increasing demand. Waiting times for treatments can stretch from weeks to months, and even years, making people feel like they're in a glacially-paced queue rather than a life-and-death race for health.

Accessibility isn't just about long waiting times. It's also about who gets access. Rural areas often find themselves at the mercy of decaying infrastructure and a severe shortage of healthcare professionals. Telemedicine had promised to bridge this gap, but it's more of a patch than a cure. Add to this the mind-numbing bureaucracy involved in simply booking an appointment, and you'll start to understand why many are clamouring for change.

Ah, bureaucracy! The unwieldy juggernaut that seems to grow tentacles overnight, each one holding a different form for you to fill out. The administrative burden on healthcare providers takes away precious time better spent on patient care. Doctors end up as reluctant paper pushers, drowning in a sea of redundant paperwork. Data entry, compliance, billing—it's a labyrinthine process that turns hospital corridors into veritable mazes, ready to entrap the unwary.

Error management is another beast entirely. Medical errors are alarmingly common and often result from miscommunication, fatigue, or simply human error. These mistakes can be as small as a misplaced decimal in a medication dosage to something as catastrophic as a wrong-site surgery. Training and protocols exist to minimise these mistakes, but the system is far from foolproof. The sad reality is that a single slip-up can have life-or-death consequences.

The diversity of health records is akin to herding cats—electronic health records (EHRs) are supposed to streamline this mess, but they often wind up adding another layer of complexity. Different healthcare providers use different systems, leading to fragmented patient data. Interoperability remains a pipe dream; transferring records from one provider to another is more like trading secrets between ancient armies rather than just clicking a button.

Data privacy and security cast a long, ominous shadow over all these challenges. With the rise of digital health records comes the inevitable rise of cyber threats. Hospitals often find themselves on the front lines of cyber-attacks, from data breaches to ransomware. The compromise of patient data isn't just a breach of trust; it's a potential death sentence if critical information falls into the wrong hands. Add GDPR to the mix, and you've got a recipe for perpetual anxiety among healthcare administrators.

Oh, and let's not forget about healthcare costs. They're eye-watering, to put it mildly. Budget constraints mean that many hospitals function more like shoestring operations rather than high-tech medical centres. Cutting-edge technologies often remain inaccessible due to prohibitively high costs. It's a Sisyphean task to balance the latest advancements in medical technology with the grim realities of budget limitations.

Supply chain issues aren't doing anyone any favours either. The pandemic exposed just how fragile our medical supply chains are. Shortages of essential medical supplies—masks, gloves, ventilators— became the norm, creating chaos that levels even the calmest of professionals. Inventory management is anything but straightforward, often resulting in either wastage or detrimental shortages.

Another critical area that needs attention is medical research. While research is the cornerstone of medical advancements, its funding is often inconsistent. Many groundbreaking studies languish due to lack of funds, trapped in a limbo of good intentions and financial constraints. The slow trickle of grants and donations can be frustratingly insufficient for the ambitious scope of modern medical science.

The workforce itself is grappling with endemic issues of burnout and mental health. Long hours, high stress, and emotional tolls are pushing healthcare professionals to their breaking points. The industry desperately needs more hands and resources, but attracting new talent is easier said than done. Compounding this is the lack of continuous education and upskilling, making it difficult for healthcare workers to keep pace with rapidly evolving medical technologies and protocols.

Accessibility to cutting-edge treatments is another thorn in the sector's side. Many patients find themselves unable to access the latest therapies, not due to lack of availability, but because of the labyrinth of red tape and conflicting medical guidelines. The disparity between what's possible in a lab and what's available to actual patients is often stark, leading to unnecessary suffering and poorer outcomes.

Then there's the issue of scalability in public health initiatives. National healthcare systems face an uphill battle in trying to implement large-scale preventive measures. Vaccination programs, health screenings, and public health campaigns often sputter out due to logistical nightmares or lack of public engagement. The ad hoc nature of these efforts means that they can be inconsistent and less impactful than intended.

As if these weren't enough, cultural and institutional resistance to change remains a persistent thorn. The reluctance to adopt new technologies or methodologies can be baffling but is often rooted in a mix of tradition, fear of the unknown, and lack of training. Changing such deeply ingrained institutional habits feels like steering a massive, rusted ship through a treacherous reef.

A final wrench in the works is the sheer unpredictability of future health crises. If the COVID-19 pandemic taught us anything, it's that we cannot predict the next curveball Mother Nature will throw at us. Preparedness remains perpetually inadequate, and the reactive nature of our systems means that we're often one step behind. This leaves a gaping vulnerability that can turn a manageable crisis into a full-blown catastrophe.

- Access to care and long waiting times
- Rural health disparities

- Bureaucratic inefficiencies

- High incidence of medical errors

- Interoperability of electronic health records

- Data privacy and cybersecurity threats

- Sky-high healthcare costs and budget constraints

- Fragile medical supply chains

- Inconsistent funding for medical research

- Workforce burnout and mental health issues

- Accessibility to modern treatments

- Difficulty in scaling public health initiatives

- Cultural and institutional resistance to change

- Unpredictability of future health crises

The NHS in particular seems to embody all these challenges rolled into one colossal enigma. Balancing the ideals of free healthcare with the ground realities of funding and operations often feels like trying to outsmart AI. Solutions are on the horizon, and technological advancements promise to ease many of these pain points, but until those are fully realised, the existing challenges remain daunting, demanding urgent and innovative responses.

Opportunities for Improvement

Given the myriad of challenges currently plaguing the healthcare sector, it's no surprise that opportunities for enhancement lie aplenty. Starting with patient care, the focus isn't just on treating ailments but on holistic wellness. There's a growing recognition that our current healthcare model often falls short in these areas, but the good news is that the solutions are tangible and within reach.

For one, technology can immensely bolster diagnostic accuracy. Picture this: utilising AI algorithms that can scrutinise medical images faster and with greater precision than a human. This isn't sci-fi; it's plausibly the next step in revolutionising medical diagnosis. Imagine the reduction in misdiagnosed cases and the speed at which patients can commence their treatment plans.

Then there's the issue of personalisation—or the lack thereof—within treatment plans. The current state sees many patients receiving a one-size-fits-all approach to medicine, which sometimes yields less than optimal outcomes. Opportunities abound in circumventing this through personalised medicine powered by AI. By analysing genetic data, AI can craft bespoke treatment plans aligning more accurately with individual patient profiles.

However, moving beyond treatments, administrative inefficiencies also cry out for reform. Anyone who's spent hours filling out forms or waiting in line can attest to how archaic some healthcare systems feel. AI-driven automation holds the key to streamlining these processes. Hospitals can optimise resource allocation, manage patient flow more effectively, and drastically reduce waiting times through predictive analytics and intelligent scheduling systems.

- **Resource Allocation:** Smart systems can ensure that resources are directed precisely where they are needed the most.

- **Administrative Tasks:** Automating administrative tasks like appointment scheduling, billing, and patient records management can free up human resources to focus more on patient care.

Additionally, telemedicine stands out as a prominent area for growth. While virtual consultations have already become more prevalent, the scope for enhancing remote patient monitoring is immense. Picture wearable devices that could track a patient's vitals in real-time and alert healthcare providers to any anomalies instantly, facilitating timely interventions. This could be particularly transformative in managing chronic diseases and in elderly care.

But let's not forget that there's a human element to healthcare that can't be wholly supplanted by even the most advanced technology. AI can assist, augment, and enhance, but it can't replace the empathy and nuanced care that human professionals provide. Therefore, a significant opportunity lies in training healthcare professionals to effectively use these advanced tools. Ensuring that they are comfortable and proficient with AI technologies will be paramount to integrating these improvements seamlessly into existing workflows.

Training programs and continuous education within medical curriculums can ensure that the coming generations of doctors and nurses are well-equipped to leverage AI in their practice. This isn't about replacing jobs, but rather about transforming roles to harness the best of both worlds: human empathy and technological precision.

Ethical considerations also warrant attention. The implementation of AI must be accompanied by robust frameworks that address data privacy and security. It's one thing to have technology capable of parsing through vast amounts of patient data, but quite another to ensure that this data is kept secure and used ethically.

Certainly, integrating AI into healthcare isn't without its challenges. However, the potential rewards—in terms of efficiency, accuracy, and patient satisfaction—are too substantial to ignore. Strategic, well-thought-out implementations can overcome hurdles such as data silos, resistance to change, and regulatory compliance issues.

In summary, there's no dearth of opportunities for improvement in the healthcare industry, especially through the integration of sophisticated AI technologies. Whether it's through increased diagnostic accuracy, personalised treatment plans, efficient administration, or enhanced patient engagement, the future of healthcare holds never-before-imagined promise. The journey towards realising these improvements might be laden with challenges, but the potential advancements usher in a transformative era, setting a gold standard in patient care and operational efficiency.

Chapter 3:
AI Innovations in Diagnosing Diseases

As we wallow in an era where the extraordinary has become the norm, the marriage of artificial intelligence and disease diagnosis stands as a testament to human ingenuity. Leveraging machine learning in imaging, hospitals are now boasting diagnostic accuracy that rivals, and sometimes even surpasses, that of seasoned radiologists. Predictive analytics is swooping in like a tech-savvy fortune teller, forecasting diseases with a precision that borders on the uncanny, allowing for early intervention and treatment. While this might sound like something plucked from the pages of a science fiction novel, it's the burgeoning reality of modern medicine. The integration of AI isn't just enhancing diagnostic tools; it's reshaping the very fabric of healthcare, turning what was once reactive care into a proactive frontier.

Machine Learning in Imaging

When we think of *artificial intelligence* infiltrating the world of healthcare, it's hard to overlook the revolutionary impact machine learning (ML) has had on medical imaging. This isn't just science fiction anymore—it's a very tangible reality in clinical settings around the globe. From X-rays to MRIs, machine learning algorithms have begun to scrutinise medical images with a level of precision that is rapidly catching up to, and in some instances surpassing, human expertise.

At its core, machine learning in imaging enables computer systems to interpret complex visual data through pattern recognition. In medical imaging, this means identifying anomalies that could signify early stages of diseases like cancer or heart disease. What used to take radiologists hours or even days to analyse can now be processed within minutes, thanks to high-powered algorithms trained on enormous datasets.

This isn't to say radiologists are going out of style; rather, they're getting an AI assistant that'll make their job more efficient. Algorithms trained on millions of images gain a level of pattern-recognition that is difficult for a single human mind to match. And because these machines never tire, they can process a practically unlimited number of images with consistent quality. Consequently, the integration of ML in imaging offers a potential lifeline in situations where radiologist shortages prevail, which are becoming increasingly common in resource-strapped healthcare systems.

The real magic, though, lies in the capabilities we're still just beginning to tap into. Imagine a scenario where an AI system isn't just identifying whether or not an image shows signs of disease, but also suggesting the best course of action based on historical data. We're talking about a future where your MRI scan doesn't just end up in a database but is actively used to tailor your treatment plan in real-time. The fusion of ML algorithms with imaging data brings personalised medicine closer than ever before.

However, the widespread implementation of these technologies isn't without its hurdles. The need for high-quality, annotated datasets is paramount. Training an algorithm requires a vast amount of information, painstakingly labelled by human experts. For disorders that are less common, acquiring such datasets can be a staggering challenge. Additionally, the ethical concerns around data privacy loom large. The granularity of medical images makes anonymising them an intricate task, one that must be tackled with both clinical and ethical rigour.

Despite these challenges, the landscape is ripe with potential, and some fascinating applications of machine learning in medical imaging are already making waves. A standout example is the role of ML in early cancer detection, especially in cancers that are notoriously difficult to diagnose at an early stage, such as pancreatic and ovarian cancer. Machine learning models trained on thousands of biopsy images are now able to identify cancerous cells with a degree of accuracy that rivals seasoned pathologists.

There's also the increasing role of ML in cardiology. Cardiac imaging is crucial for diagnosing heart diseases, which remain a leading cause of death worldwide. Machine learning models can analyse echocardiograms and cardiac MRIs to detect abnormalities like ejection fractions or myocardial infarctions. The speed and accuracy provided by these models can be the difference between life and death, as quicker diagnosis often results in more effective interventions.

Diabetes management has also seen noteworthy advances with the application of machine learning. Diabetic retinopathy, a condition that can lead to blindness if not detected early, is becoming easier to manage with automated image analysis of retinal scans. By flagging problematic areas and suggesting treatment protocols, ML is making regular screening more efficient and cost-effective, thereby reducing the chances of severe complications.

Let's not forget the more everyday applications that make a world of difference, particularly in developing countries. Portable ultrasound devices paired with ML algorithms enable healthcare workers in remote areas to diagnose conditions on the spot. In places where access to specialised medical care is limited, this technology can be a game-changer.

It would be remiss not to mention the impact of deep learning, a subfield of ML, which uses neural networks to mimic the human brain. Convolutional neural networks (CNNs), in particular, have shown tremendous promise in image recognition tasks. These algorithms have become proficient in tasks as varied as skin lesion classification and fracture detection in orthopaedics. Moreover, the use of CNNs richly augments the capabilities of ML models, pushing the boundaries of what's possible in image-based diagnostics.

Clinical trials and extensive research validate these algorithms, ensuring they undergo rigorous testing before making their way into hospitals. Regulatory bodies like the FDA (Food and Drug Administration) in the US and MHRA (Medicines and Healthcare Products Regulatory Agency) in the UK are increasingly focused on creating frameworks that allow for the seamless integration of AI into medical practices without compromising patient safety.

In conclusion, machine learning in imaging marks a poignant leap forward in the intersection of technology and healthcare. Far from being just another feature in the proverbial Swiss army knife of AI innovations, it stands as a monumental pillar holding up the future of diagnostics. Be prepared to see more of these intelligent systems peppering through medical practices worldwide, not only enhancing the accuracy and speed of diagnoses but also profoundly influencing treatment pathways. In the realm of healthcare, where every second counts, machine learning could very well be the key to saving countless lives.

Case Studies and Examples serve as the crucibles where theoretical advancements are tested against the harsh reality of healthcare's complexities. In the vast landscape of AI innovations, few areas are more promising and simultaneously challenging than the application of machine learning in imaging. Through a series of compelling case studies, we can see how these technologies are not just pie-in-the-sky fantasies, but real-world solutions with tangible benefits. Let's dive into a few examples to illustrate this.

First up, consider the work being done at Stanford University in the United States, where researchers developed an AI algorithm to detect pneumonia from chest X-rays. Before their innovation, diagnosing pneumonia involved a radiologist painstakingly examining images, a process prone to human error and limited by the availability of specialised professionals. The Stanford algorithm, however, leverages deep learning techniques to outperform radiologists in identifying pneumonia. By training on thousands of X-rays, the system became adept at spotting the tell-tale signs of pneumonia, often invisible to the untrained eye. What's particularly interesting is the algorithm's ability to learn and adapt; as more data is fed into the system, its diagnostic accuracy improves, promising a future where misdiagnosis rates plummet.

Another fascinating example hails from the Moorfields Eye Hospital in London, which teamed up with Google DeepMind to address the burgeoning issue of macular degeneration, a leading cause of blindness. By using a dataset comprising eye scans, DeepMind's AI was trained to detect signs of macular degeneration with an accuracy level matching that of the top ophthalmologists. The AI doesn't just stop at diagnosis; it also recommends the most appropriate course of treatment, which is critical in conditions where early intervention can save a person's sight. The marriage of AI and ophthalmology in this case exemplifies the dual benefits of enhanced diagnostic precision and improved patient outcomes.

In the realm of cancer detection, the University of Edinburgh has been making strides with an AI system designed to catch early signs of colorectal cancer. This particular cancer is notoriously difficult to detect in its initial stages, often leading to late diagnoses and poor prognoses. The AI system scans colonoscopy images, looking for abnormal growths and polyps that are easily missed by human eyes. The system's real triumph, however, isn't just in detection. It also analyses the growth patterns and cellular structures of these anomalies, providing invaluable insights into whether they are likely to be benign or malignant. This granular level of detail equips oncologists with the information they need to make better-informed decisions, potentially increasing survival rates.

Then we have the example of AI in dermatology. SkinVision, a Dutch company, created a mobile app leveraging AI to screen for skin cancer. Users can take photos of their skin lesions and upload them to the app. The AI analyses these images to determine the likelihood that a lesion is malignant. This technology democratizes access to early-stage screening, especially in regions where dermatologists are scarce. It's a blend of convenience and cutting-edge technology that empowers individuals to take control of their health in unprecedented ways. The app's accuracy has been validated in clinical settings, and it has already identified numerous cases of melanoma, underscoring its life-saving potential.

A rather sobering yet inspiring case comes from India, where early-stage breast cancer detection is a considerable challenge due to limited healthcare infrastructure. Niramai, an AI-driven health tech company, developed a non-invasive, radiation-free method for early breast cancer screening using thermal imaging and machine learning algorithms. This low-cost solution is revolutionary for a country where many women lack access to traditional mammograms. Niramai's approach uses thermal sensors to measure temperature variations on the skin's surface, which are analysed by an AI to detect cancerous growths. This method has shown promise not only in improving diagnostic accuracy but also in making cancer screening accessible to a broader population.

On the operational side, consider the use of AI to optimise workforces in hospitals. Take University Hospital in Zurich, which piloted a system to streamline its nursing staff schedules. Using machine learning, the AI forecasts patient influx and adjusts staffing levels accordingly, ensuring that the hospital always operates at optimal efficiency. This isn't just about cost-cutting; it's about better quality care. Nurses are less overworked, leading to fewer mistakes and improved patient satisfaction. It's also worth noting that the implementation of this system led to a surprising reduction in operation costs, which could be redirected towards patient care and other crucial areas.

Resource allocation, another critical component of hospital management, has seen significant improvement with AI. In Cedars-Sinai Medical Center in Los Angeles, an AI-driven tool aids in the allocation of resources such as ICU beds and ventilators. By analysing a combination of patient data and historical trends, this AI can predict which patients are most likely to need intensive care. This means that resources are prepped and ready before they're even required, effectively reducing wait times and improving outcomes during critical periods, such as the peaks of the COVID-19 pandemic.

The administrative tasks that bog down healthcare workers are also getting a tech overhaul. In a case study from Beth Israel Deaconess Medical Center in Boston, a natural language processing (NLP) system was implemented to assist with the documentation workload. This AI listens to doctor-patient interactions and automatically fills out electronic health records (EHRs), freeing up clinicians to spend more time with patients and less time on paperwork. Not only does this improve the patient experience, but it also reduces the rates of burnout among healthcare professionals. Furthermore, the AI system has demonstrated exceptional accuracy, capturing subtleties in medical conversations that even human scribes might miss.

Shifting focus to patient engagement, we find AI chatbots and virtual consultations playing a transformative role. Babylon Health in the UK offers a prime example. Their AI-powered chatbot can triage health queries, provide medical information, and even schedule consultations with human doctors if needed. This system has alleviated some of the pressure on the NHS, allowing overburdened clinicians to focus on more severe cases. It's an elegant solution to the age-old problem of limited access to healthcare services, particularly beneficial in rural or remote areas where medical practitioners are scarce. The chatbot employs natural language processing to understand and respond to a wide range of patient queries, making it a versatile tool in the healthcare ecosystem.

Then there is the intriguing development in wearable technology, as exemplified by the partnership between Fitbit and Google. Wearable devices now go beyond tracking steps to monitor vital signs like heart rate, sleep patterns, and even glucose levels in diabetics. AI algorithms analyse this constant stream of data, flagging any abnormalities for medical review. Take, for instance, the case of John, who received an early warning about atrial fibrillation symptoms through his smartwatch's AI. The alert prompted him to seek medical advice, potentially saving him from a stroke. This kind of real-time health monitoring transforms not just patient care but also the nature of the doctor-patient relationship, making it more proactive than reactive.

Predictive Analytics for Early Detection

Imagine catching a disease before it even shows symptoms, nipping potential health crises in the bud. That's not some futuristic sci-fi scenario; it's precisely what predictive analytics aims to do. At its core, this technology analyses vast amounts of data to forecast health issues before they escalate. Think of it as a crystal ball that uses numbers and algorithms instead of mystic smoke. Predictive analytics is quickly becoming a cornerstone of AI innovations in diagnosing diseases.

The power behind this approach lies in data—massive volumes of it, mind you. Hospitals, clinics, and even wearable devices generate mountains of data every day. Patient records, lifestyle information, genetic sequences, you name it. By leveraging machine learning algorithms and AI models, healthcare professionals can sift through these data points to identify patterns that even a trained eye might miss. This isn't just about being one step ahead; it's about being leagues ahead.

Consider chronic diseases like diabetes and heart disease. These conditions often have subtle, early indicators that can be detected through proper data analysis. AI systems can monitor patients in real-time, alerting healthcare providers to any anomalies that suggest the onset of these diseases. For instance, fluctuations in blood sugar levels or unusual heart rate patterns picked up by wearable technology can be flagged and addressed before they become critical issues.

Moreover, the integration of social determinants of health into predictive models is setting new standards. Factors such as socioeconomic status, geography, and lifestyle choices are now being woven into the algorithms. Imagine an AI system that considers not just your medical history but also your occupation, living conditions, and even your grocery shopping habits. The level of personalisation doesn't just stop at genetic data but extends to granular aspects of daily life, offering a more holistic view of one's health.

The use of predictive analytics also shines brightly in the field of oncology. Early detection of cancer can significantly improve survival rates, and AI tools are making this a reality. By analysing medical imaging, genetic information, and even biopsy reports, AI systems can predict the likelihood of cancer development. This leads to earlier interventions, often before a tumour has the chance to spread. It's a significant leap forward from traditional methods where diagnosis often occurs only after symptoms appear.

However, like any new technology, predictive analytics is not without its challenges. It's vital for models to be trained with diverse datasets to avoid biases. For instance, algorithms trained mainly on data from Western populations might not perform as well in diagnosing diseases among different ethnic groups. It is paramount to ensure inclusivity in the datasets to make predictive analytics universally reliable.

Despite these challenges, several success stories showcase the potential of predictive analytics. One notable example is the collaborative effort between tech giants and leading hospitals to develop predictive models for sepsis—an ailment notorious for its rapid onset and high mortality rate. Early identification of sepsis can save countless lives, and predictive analytics tools have shown promising results in flagging potential cases before they reach critical stages. Hospitals employing these tools report faster response times and more effective treatments.

Let's not forget the cost implications. Predictive analytics has the potential to save significant amounts of money for healthcare systems. By identifying diseases early, treatment can be less invasive, less costly, and more effective. It reduces the need for prolonged hospital stays, expensive surgeries, and extensive recovery periods. In a world where healthcare budgets are always under scrutiny, this technology offers a rare opportunity to cut costs while improving patient outcomes.

The world of mental health can also benefit hugely from predictive analytics. Conditions such as depression and anxiety often remain undiagnosed until they have seriously impacted an individual's life. By analysing behavioural data, social media activity, and even speech patterns, AI can provide early warnings about mental health issues. It's not about replacing the human touch in therapy but ensuring timely interventions and more personalised care plans.

Governments and policymakers are increasingly noticing the potential of predictive analytics. Some national health services are already piloting AI-based programs to screen for diseases like breast cancer and diabetes. These initiatives are proving successful, prompting further investments and strategic planning to integrate predictive analytics on a larger scale. The idea is to move from reactive to proactive healthcare systems, fundamentally shifting how public health is managed.

Still, implementing such technologies requires addressing several legal and ethical considerations. Data privacy remains a top concern. Sensitive health data should be handled with the utmost care to ensure patient confidentiality. Transparent algorithms that can be reviewed and audited by independent bodies are essential to maintain trust in these systems. There's also the question of accountability—if a predictive model fails, who bears the responsibility? These are complex issues that regulators, technologists, and healthcare providers must tackle collaboratively.

Finally, it's crucial to bring healthcare professionals on board. Predictive analytics requires a shift in mindset from traditional diagnostic methods to data-driven approaches. Training and education programs are essential to equip medical staff with the skills needed to effectively use these new tools. Encouragingly, many medical schools are already integrating data science and AI into their curriculums, preparing the next generation of healthcare providers for an AI-augmented future.

In summary, predictive analytics is poised to revolutionise early disease detection. With its ability to analyse vast amounts of data, identify patterns, and offer personalised insights, it's transforming how we approach healthcare. From oncology to mental health, this technology is paving the way for early interventions and better outcomes. Yes, there are challenges to overcome, but the potential benefits far outweigh the hurdles. The future of healthcare isn't just about treating illnesses; it's about preventing them before they even begin. And that's a game-changer in every sense.

Chapter 4:
Personalised Medicine and Treatment Plans

The era of one-size-fits-all healthcare is swiftly giving way to a more tailored approach, all thanks to personalised medicine and treatment plans. Picture a future where treatments aren't generic prescriptions, but carefully crafted strategies based on your unique genetic makeup, lifestyle, and even your microbiome. This paradigm shift is largely driven by AI-driven genomics, enabling the identification of genetic markers that can predict disease susceptibility and treatment responses with uncanny precision. It's like swapping a sledgehammer for a scalpel. Not only does this promise to enhance treatment efficacy, but it also minimizes adverse effects, making healthcare more efficient and patient-friendly. Undoubtedly, we're stepping into a world where healthcare is not just about treating the disease but about understanding and treating the individual at a molecular level.

AI-Driven Genomics

The healthcare sector is on the cusp of an extraordinary transformation, and it's largely being powered by Artificial Intelligence (AI). Among the most revolutionary areas of AI application is genomics, a field that is foundational to personalised medicine and treatment plans. AI-driven genomics refers to the use of sophisticated algorithms and machine learning models to analyse massive datasets of genetic information. The aim? To develop tailor-made healthcare solutions that cater to an individual's unique genetic makeup. Let's dive into the magic of this confluence of AI and genomics.

Genomics itself is a relatively young science, but one that has grown at an astronomical pace. Once a laborious and costly endeavour, sequencing the human genome has now become quicker, cheaper, and more accessible. Thanks to advancements in next-generation sequencing technologies, the process that used to take years and billions of dollars can now be done in days for a fraction of the cost. However, the real game-changer has been AI, which has unlocked the potential lying dormant in terabytes of genomic data.

One of the primary ways AI is utilised in genomics is through predictive modelling. AI algorithms can identify patterns in genetic data that may correlate with specific diseases or health conditions. These models can predict a person's susceptibility to various ailments, from common disorders like diabetes to rare genetic conditions. For instance, how can AI predict whether you'll develop Alzheimer's in later years? By sifting through a labyrinth of genetic markers and lifestyle factors—something that is virtually impossible for humans to do with the same speed and accuracy.

Consider the BRCA1 and BRCA2 genes, mutations of which are associated with a higher risk of breast and ovarian cancer. AI can analyse these genes and flag mutations that might go unnoticed in traditional genetic testing, giving healthcare providers the insight needed to recommend preventive measures well before the onset of disease.

AI-driven genomics can also play a critical role in pharmacogenomics, which focuses on how genes affect a person's response to drugs. This is crucial because a drug that works wonders for one patient might be completely ineffective or even harmful to another. AI algorithms can analyse the genetic factors that influence drug metabolism, resistance, or toxicity, enabling clinicians to prescribe the most effective medication with the least side effects for each patient. In other words, it brings us closer to the holy grail of medicine: the right treatment, for the right patient, at the right time.

Moreover, let's not overlook the essential part AI can play in gene editing and CRISPR technology. With its ability to analyse vast data sets and simulate billions of genetic variations, AI can significantly enhance the precision and safety of gene-editing techniques. This has promising implications for treating genetic disorders like cystic fibrosis or muscular dystrophy, diseases that, until now, have had limited treatment options.

But we must remember, this isn't a sci-fi utopia where AI takes over entirely. Human expertise remains irreplaceable. AI aids geneticists and healthcare providers by offering data-driven insights, identifying previously overlooked genetic markers, and suggesting possible treatment pathways. The final call, however, is made by skilled practitioners who interpret AI's findings in the context of a patient's overall health and lifestyle.

AI's role doesn't stop at identifying genetic risks; it also encompasses developing personalised treatment plans. Imagine a world where the treatment protocol for cancer patients is tailored to their genetic makeup. AI algorithms, trained on thousands of genomic datasets, can suggest bespoke treatment strategies, minimising side effects and maximising efficacy. Clinical trials, often a cumbersome and lengthy process, can also benefit from AI by identifying the right candidates and accelerating the trial phases, bringing new drugs to market faster than ever before.

The broader implications for public health are equally staggering. When utilised on a population level, AI can predict genetic susceptibility to various diseases, allowing for more effective screening programs and preventive healthcare strategies. Public health policies can be shaped based on genetic trends, which, in turn, could lead to a healthier population and reduced healthcare costs. It's a win-win.

However, like any powerful technology, AI-driven genomics comes with its own set of challenges. One pressing issue is data privacy and security. Genetic data is extremely sensitive, and any breach could have significant repercussions. Ensuring robust data protection mechanisms is, therefore, of paramount importance. Ethical considerations also abound—questions about consent, data ownership, and the potential for genetic discrimination need to be carefully navigated.

Moreover, AI algorithms are not infallible. They can be biased, especially if trained on non-diverse datasets. To prevent skewed results, it is vital to train AI systems on varied genetic data that includes different ethnicities and demographic backgrounds. This would ensure that personalised medicine is truly inclusive and beneficial for all, rather than a select few.

Let's not forget the importance of interdisciplinary collaboration in this innovative field. Geneticists, data scientists, bioinformaticians, and healthcare practitioners must work together to harness the full potential of AI-driven genomics. This symbiotic relationship is crucial for translating genetic insights into tangible healthcare solutions. Furthermore, as AI technologies continue to advance, the need for ongoing training and education for healthcare professionals becomes even more critical, ensuring they can leverage these tools effectively and ethically.

In conclusion, AI-driven genomics stands as a formidable pillar supporting the edifice of personalised medicine. By leveraging the computational prowess of AI, the intricacies of the human genome are being unravelled at an unprecedented rate. This not only opens up new avenues for diagnosing and treating diseases but also heralds a new era of preventative healthcare. While challenges persist, the potential benefits far outweigh the hurdles. AI-driven genomics promises a future where medicine is not just a blanket solution but a carefully woven tapestry, designed uniquely for each one of us. That, perhaps, is the most exciting change awaiting the healthcare sector.

Tailoring Treatments to Individual Patients

Health is a deeply personal affair. What works wonders for one person could be utterly ineffective for another. This has been the challenge in healthcare for centuries—juggling the complexities of unique human biology with the need for general approaches in treatment. Fortunately, the tide is turning. Thanks to advancements in AI and genomics, we're stepping into a new era where treatments can be finely tailored to individual patients. This isn't science fiction; it's the new reality we've been waiting for.

The application of AI in personalising treatment plans begins with data. Mountains of it. We're talking genetic data, lifestyle information, medical history, and even social determinants of health. By feeding this data into sophisticated AI algorithms, healthcare professionals can detect patterns and make predictions about which treatments are most likely to work for a specific individual. It's like having an ultra-smart personal assistant who's read every medical journal, knows your entire medical history, and understands your unique genetic makeup.

One practical application of AI is in pharmacogenomics—the study of how genes affect a person's response to drugs. Imagine you're prescribed a new medication: rather than enduring the frustrating trial-and-error process, your healthcare provider can perform genetic testing and use AI to predict how you will respond to different medications. They can then select the drug that's most likely to work for you, minimising side effects and maximising efficacy. It's precision medicine at its finest.

The power of AI in tailoring treatments isn't just limited to pharmacology. AI's predictive capabilities can be a game-changer in chronic disease management as well. Conditions like diabetes, heart disease, and asthma require ongoing management, and what works well at one stage of life might not be effective later on. AI algorithms can analyse continuous streams of data from wearable devices and electronic health records to adjust treatment plans in real time, ensuring that they're always aligned with the patient's current condition.

Consider the realm of cancer treatment. Oncology has seen some of the most promising developments in tailored treatments. Traditional cancer treatments can be something of a blunt instrument—effective, yes, but often with significant side effects. Now, AI is making it possible to devise personalised treatment plans that target the unique genetic mutations within an individual's cancer cells. By sequencing the genome of a tumour, AI can help identify which treatments will be most effective, thereby increasing the chances of success and sparing the patient from unnecessary side effects. It's like replacing a sledgehammer with a scalpel.

Another compelling application is in the field of mental health. Treating mental health conditions has always been fraught with challenges, partly because what works for one mind may be entirely unsuitable for another. AI can help decode the complexities of the human brain, identifying nuances that might be missed by traditional diagnostic methods. By analysing data from brain scans, clinical records, and even patient-reported outcomes, AI can assist clinicians in designing more effective, personalised treatment plans for conditions such as depression, anxiety, and schizophrenia.

AI's role in tailoring treatments extends beyond medicine itself to patient behaviour and lifestyle. We know that lifestyle factors like diet, exercise, and sleep have a profound impact on health outcomes. AI can help patients make informed decisions about their lifestyles by providing personalised recommendations based on a comprehensive analysis of their unique data. For instance, a patient with high blood pressure might receive tailored advice on dietary changes, stress management techniques, and exercise routines that are most likely to benefit them, considering their genetic predispositions and health history. This approach moves us away from generic advice towards actionable, personalised guidelines that can significantly improve health outcomes.

Personalising treatments also involves looking at the whole patient, not just their medical conditions. Socioeconomic factors, cultural background, and even personal preferences can influence how a treatment plan is received and adhered to. AI can help capture this wider context and use it to tailor interventions. For example, a patient's work schedule or family responsibilities might affect their ability to follow a particular treatment plan. By integrating this kind of data, AI can assist in designing plans that are not only medically effective but also practically feasible for the patient.

Ethical considerations naturally arise when dealing with such highly personal data. Consent, privacy, and data security are paramount. If we're to gather detailed personal information—including genetic data—patients need to trust that their information will be handled with the utmost care and confidentiality. Health systems must therefore be transparent about how data is used and stored. Complex algorithms also need rigorous validation to ensure that they're accurate and free from biases. These concerns are not trivial, but they are manageable with careful governance and ethical oversight.

The gradual shift towards personalised treatment can also alleviate some of the pressure on healthcare systems. By allocating resources more efficiently and reducing unnecessary treatments, personalised medicine has the potential to make healthcare more sustainable. For instance, predictive analytics can help identify patients who are at high risk of hospital readmission and intervene preemptively, improving patient outcomes and reducing the financial burden on healthcare systems.

Moreover, the integration of AI in personalising treatments can significantly improve patient satisfaction and engagement. Patients are more likely to comply with treatment plans that are specifically designed for them. When people see that their care is tailored to their needs and preferences, it fosters a sense of involvement and trust in the healthcare process. This, in turn, can lead to better health outcomes and improved quality of life.

In summary, tailoring treatments to individual patients is not just a visionary concept but an increasingly practical reality. Thanks to AI, healthcare is inching towards a future where treatments are as unique as the people receiving them. From genetic profiling to lifestyle recommendations and proactive chronic disease management, AI is poised to revolutionise how we approach patient care. As we continue to navigate the ethical and logistical challenges, one thing is clear: the era of one-size-fits-all medical care is drawing to a close. And not a moment too soon.

Chapter 5:
AI in Healthcare Operations

While the spotlight often shines on AI's potential to revolutionise diagnostics and treatment, a quieter yet equally transformative wave is making its mark on healthcare operations. AI is optimising hospital management by enhancing everything from resource allocation to streamlining administrative tasks. Picture algorithms that can predict patient admissions, ensuring bed availability and reducing wait times. Robotic process automation (RPA) is tackling the mundane but necessary paperwork, allowing healthcare staff to focus on patient care rather than drowning in forms. It's like a backstage crew working tirelessly so the show can go on without a hitch, albeit with fewer human errors and far more efficiency. The NHS and global health systems alike are keenly eyeing these developments, aiming to strike a balance between cutting costs and improving patient outcomes. The mundane is being digitised so the extraordinary can flourish, turning administrative burdens into streamlined, efficient processes.

Optimising Hospital Management

How do you put out fires before they start? No, this isn't a manual for firefighters, but it's pretty close when it comes to hospital management. With the staggering complexity and ceaseless activity of modern hospitals, operational efficiency isn't a luxury but a necessity. And that's where our hero, Artificial Intelligence (AI), swoops in, cape fluttering. AI is revolutionising the healthcare sector by making hospital management not just manageable but optimised to a breath-taking degree.

At the heart of hospital management lies resource allocation. It's a juggling act of epic proportions. Beds, medical staff, equipment, and even time need to be allocated with precision. Here's where AI flexes its algorithmic muscles. By analysing vast datasets, AI can predict patient admissions, discharges, and even potential emergencies with uncanny accuracy. This foresight allows hospitals to allocate resources in advance, ensuring that the right number of staff and equipment are available when needed. It's like having a crystal ball, but grounded in data rather than mysticism.

Consider a scenario where a hospital is facing an influx of patients due to a seasonal flu outbreak. Traditionally, this would cause chaos, with overbooked consultations, equipment shortages, and overworked staff. Enter AI, and suddenly it's a different story. Predictive algorithms can analyse past data to forecast demand spikes, thus allowing administrators to pre-emptively increase staff rosters, stockpile essential medications, and ensure equipment is in place. The result? A smoother operation that mitigates chaos and maintains quality care.

Navigating the labyrinth of administrative tasks is another area where AI shines. Hospitals churn out mountains of paperwork every single day, encompassing patient records, billing information, and compliance documentation. Manually managing these papers is not only time-consuming but also error-prone. AI algorithms can automate these tasks, freeing up human staff to focus on patient care. Imagine an AI system that can scan, sort, and file documents at lightning speed. No more clerical errors, lost files, or frazzled admin staff.

In addition to automating routine tasks, AI can also streamline complex administrative processes like scheduling. With doctors juggling multiple roles and unpredictable patient needs, creating schedules that optimise staff availability and patient care can be a nightmare. AI-driven scheduling tools can analyse multiple variables— such as doctor availability, patient needs, and even room availability— to create the most efficient schedules. It can even accommodate last-minute changes with ease, ensuring that everyone is in the right place at the right time.

But don't think it's all just about the inner workings of hospitals. AI's impact extends to the patient experience as well. Imagine a world where checking into a hospital is as seamless as scanning your boarding pass at an airport kiosk. Self-service AI stations can handle check-ins, update patient records, and even direct patients to the correct department. This not only reduces wait times but also relieves the burden on front-line staff, who can then focus on more critical tasks.

Another mundane yet critical task AI can address is inventory management. Hospitals must continuously monitor and manage countless medical supplies, from mundane bandages to high-tech diagnostic machines. Running out of essential supplies can be disastrous. AI can scrutinise usage patterns and predict when supplies are running low, automatically placing orders to replenish stocks before a shortage occurs. This not only ensures that critical supplies are always available but also optimises inventory costs.

However, it's not all smooth sailing. The implementation of AI in hospital management comes with its own set of challenges. For instance, how do you integrate these sophisticated systems into existing workflows without causing disruption? It's a bit like trying to change the wheels on a moving car. Successful integration requires careful planning, training for staff, and ongoing support to address any issues that arise. Moreover, data privacy and security become paramount concerns when dealing with sensitive patient information. Robust security measures must be in place to protect data from breaches or misuse.

Despite these hurdles, the benefits far outweigh the challenges. AI has the potential to make hospital management more proactive rather than reactive. By anticipating needs and streamlining processes, AI allows hospitals to focus on their core mission: delivering high-quality patient care. This not only improves patient outcomes but also boosts staff morale by reducing burnout and administrative overload.

Moreover, the financial implications are significant. Efficient resource allocation and streamlined administrative processes can lead to substantial cost savings. These savings can then be reinvested into improving patient care, acquiring advanced medical technologies, or supporting research initiatives. It's a virtuous cycle where efficiency begets quality and vice versa.

Ultimately, AI in hospital management represents the fusion of technology and healthcare in the most practical way. It's like having an all-seeing, all-knowing assistant that tirelessly works behind the scenes to keep everything running smoothly. And as AI technologies continue to evolve, their capabilities will only expand, potentially transforming every facet of hospital operations.

So, the next time you find yourself in a hospital, take a moment to appreciate the intricate ballet of operations happening around you. Behind the scenes, AI might just be the unsung hero, orchestrating a symphony of efficiency, precision, and care.

Resource Allocation has always been a critical aspect of healthcare. As AI technologies burgeon, the age-old conundrum of optimising resources doesn't just find a fresh perspective but takes on a whole new dimension. Efficient resource allocation isn't merely about budget balancing anymore; it's about leveraging advanced algorithms to predict and allocate resources where they're needed the most.

Smarter resource allocation begins with data. Hospitals and healthcare facilities generate a vast amount of data every single day. Using AI to sift through these reams of data can unveil patterns that were previously invisible. This predictive capability allows for better planning, ensuring that resources like staff, equipment, and medicines are optimised based on actual demand rather than historical usage. Imagine a hospital that already knows it's going to need more paediatric nurses next flu season because the AI model forecasted it months in advance. Simple, right? Yet profoundly impactful.

Beyond human resources, AI-driven resource allocation extends to medical equipment. Take MRI machines, for instance—expensive, indispensable, and often in short supply. AI can help manage the schedule to ensure that these machines are used to their full capacity, reducing downtime and increasing throughput. Moreover, by analysing patient data, AI can suggest the best timings and specific uses, potentially improving patient outcomes. No longer is it just an administrative function; it's a sophisticated, dynamic balancing act.

Let's not forget the pharmaceuticals. Medication stockpiling is another area where intelligent resource allocation can revolutionise operations. AI isn't just about ordering drugs before they run out; it's about understanding trends, peak periods, and even regional disease outbreaks. With predictive analytics, it's possible to anticipate drug shortages and make preemptive purchases to mitigate risks. And in cases of unexpected spikes in demand, AI can provide alternative pathways or substitutes, ensuring that patient care is not compromised. For any facility, this is nothing short of a logistical masterstroke.

AI's predictive prowess also addresses bed allocation, which has been a thorny issue for many healthcare systems. With AI's help, hospitals can predict patient admissions and discharges with remarkable accuracy, ensuring that bed availability is optimally managed. This is particularly crucial during seasonal peaks or unforeseen epidemics. Additionally, AI can provide real-time updates, helping staff make-informed decisions swiftly.

However, it's essential to recognise that all these benefits do come with their challenges. Implementing AI systems requires significant financial investment and a shift in the organisational mindset. Staff training becomes crucial, ensuring that everyone from IT professionals to ward managers understands how to interpret and act on AI-generated data.

Resource allocation isn't just numbers and algorithms; it's about the heartbeat of a healthcare facility operating smoothly. The human element, backed by technology, will always be indispensable. As AI continues to weave its way into the fabric of healthcare, the challenge will be to balance technological advancements with the irreplaceable empathy and intuition of human professionals.

In sum, AI-driven resource allocation promises a more efficient, responsive, and financially sustainable healthcare system. Given the increasing pressures on global health services, from ageing populations to emerging diseases, this technological partnership seems not just logical but essential. It heralds a new era where resources are not just managed but anticipated, ensuring that the right person gets the right care at the right time.

Streamlining Administrative Tasks

If there is one area in healthcare that nobody romanticises, it's the administrative grind. Paperwork, scheduling, claims processing—all essential, all mundane. Thankfully, artificial intelligence (AI) is stepping in, promising to change the game entirely. The impact? You might just start seeing less harried hospital staff and smoother patient experiences. But let's dig into the specifics and find out how.

Let's start with *appointment scheduling*. Patient's non-attendances and scheduling clashes have traditionally thrown wrenches into the smooth operation of healthcare facilities. With AI, predictive algorithms can anticipate unfilled slots and suggest optimal rebooking, significantly improving efficiency. Moreover, AI-driven systems can integrate patient preferences and clinician availability to automatically generate optimized schedules. The goal? Fewer headaches and better resource utilisation. No doctor enjoys sitting idle, and no patient likes waiting weeks for an appointment. AI aims to strike a balance that keeps everyone happier.

Then there's the dreaded realm of *claims processing*. Anyone who's ever dealt with medical insurance knows the labyrinthine ordeal it can be. AI can alleviate this by automating the entire process—from claims submission to approval. Through machine learning, these systems can quickly flag errors, identify patterns of fraud, and ensure that claims comply with regulations. The upshot? Faster claim settlements and reduced administrative costs. It's like handing over the rigmarole to a hyper-efficient administrative assistant, minus the salary and tea breaks.

Here's another exciting development: **Natural Language Processing (NLP)**. With NLP, AI can sift through mountains of paperwork in mere seconds. From electronic health records to prescriptions, these systems can capture, analyse, and store data with unprecedented speed and accuracy. Imagine healthcare professionals focusing more on patient care instead of wrestling with bureaucratic bottlenecks. AI can be the oil in the cogs of administrative machinery, making processes smoother and more reliable.

Let's not overlook *inventory management*, a task as dull as it is crucial. Ensuring that supplies are well-stocked without being overstocked is a balancing act. AI can tip the scales in your favour. Predictive analytics can forecast usage patterns and suggest timely reorders. It's like having a crystal ball for your hospital's supply room. Need syringes, bandages, or that fancy new imaging equipment? Your friendly neighbourhood AI will keep tabs on everything, ensuring you're never caught off-guard.

A key area where AI is making waves is in **human resources**. Recruitment and staff management in healthcare settings can be extraordinarily complex. AI algorithms can streamline the hiring process by sifting through CVs, highlighting the most qualified candidates, and even identifying potential biases in hiring practices. Imagine a more diverse and capable workforce, all thanks to a set of well-calibrated algorithms. Once hired, managing shifts can also be a breeze with AI-driven rostering systems that take into account staff availability, skill sets, and patient needs.

Predicting patient admissions is another area where AI shines. Historical data analysis combined with real-time inputs allows AI systems to make pretty precise predictions about bed occupancy and staffing requirements. This kind of foresight is invaluable, especially during seasonal spikes in patient numbers. With the right AI tools, healthcare facilities can optimise their staffing levels, ensuring that they never find themselves short-staffed—or overstaffed, for that matter.

On a broader level, *patient data management* is getting a much-needed facelift thanks to AI. Centralised data systems powered by AI can ensure that all patient information is up-to-date, accurate, and easily accessible to authorised personnel. Integrated systems mean fewer data silos and more unified patient care. After all, when it comes to healthcare, information is power. The more seamless the data flow, the better the care patients receive.

Furthermore, **compliance** with regulatory standards is a nonstop grind for healthcare administrators. AI can simplify regulatory compliance by continuously monitoring systems for adherence to legal standards. Instead of retrospectively correcting errors, AI can provide real-time alerts, ensuring compliance before issues snowball into full-blown crises. This means fewer fines, fewer lawsuits, and a smoother operational flow overall.

Delving into the nuts and bolts of administrative tasks, we find that *billing* is a labyrinth of codes and regulations. Here, AI can categorise procedures and treatments, ensuring that billing codes are accurately applied, reducing the chances of underbilling or overbilling. Automated billing processes can significantly cut down on the financial discrepancies that plague healthcare institutions. In essence, the billing office could soon operate less like a chaotic post-Christmas sale and more like a well-oiled financial machine.

Let's not forget about patient *referrals*. Referring patients to specialists often involves stacks of paperwork and endless phone calls. AI can automate referrals, ensuring that all the necessary patient data is accurately transferred to the right specialist without any human error. This not only speeds up the referral process but also ensures that patients receive timely care without the bureaucratic delays that can exacerbate medical conditions.

The perks of AI don't stop there. Data analytics for **performance metrics** can assist administrators in tracking the efficiency of various departments. By identifying bottlenecks and inefficient practices, healthcare administrators can implement changes that drive performance improvements. AI-driven analytics can also offer predictions, providing foresight into potential future challenges and areas for growth. It's like having a strategic consultant wired directly into every facet of your operations.

The potential for AI in streamlining *communication* within healthcare facilities can't be overstated. AI systems can manage internal communication channels, ensuring that the right information reaches the right people at the right time. Whether it's alerting the ICU staff about an incoming critical case or notifying the pharmacy about a sudden spike in demand for a particular medication, AI can facilitate smooth and effective communication.

Even in the dark, often ignored corners of *facility maintenance*, AI shines brightly. Predictive maintenance algorithms can monitor the condition of medical equipment and infrastructure, predicting failures before they occur. This ensures that crucial equipment is always operational, eliminating the risk of sudden breakdowns that can jeopardise patient care. A minor glitch won't turn into a major catastrophe if an AI tells you exactly when to perform maintenance checks.

In the administration world, time and accuracy are everything, and AI is poised to be the ultimate ally in this ongoing affair with efficiency. From reducing the time doctors spend on administrative tasks to making sure that every cog in the healthcare machinery runs smoothly, AI's influence is undoubtedly transformative. The streamlining of administrative tasks isn't just a distant dream; it's fast becoming a tangible reality, reshaping how healthcare facilities around the world operate.

So, while automation and AI won't completely eradicate human errors and inefficiencies, they certainly tip the scales in favour of a more seamless, efficient healthcare system. Streamlining administrative tasks with AI isn't merely about shaving down expenses or boosting profits—though those are welcomed side effects—it's fundamentally about reclaiming time and resources that can be better spent on patient

Chapter 6:
Enhancing Patient Engagement

As we wade through the labyrinth of modern healthcare, the spotlight on patient engagement becomes brighter and impeccable. Virtual health assistants, including chatbots and virtual consultations, are no longer sci-fi whims but practical tools reshaping patient interaction and convenience. These digital confederates are revolutionising how patients access care, making it more immediate and personalised. Couple this technological wizardry with wearable tech and remote monitoring, and you've got a recipe for continuous, real-time health feedback. This shift doesn't just help in tracking vitals or chronic conditions; it fosters a proactive attitude towards one's own health. Consequently, the walls of traditional healthcare silos are crumbling, making way for a more interconnected and responsive system—where your wristband might just nudge you to schedule that much-needed check-up before the symptoms even manifest. Such advancements aren't merely incremental; they're catalysts for a patient-centred future, where engagement isn't just encouraged; it's inevitable.

Virtual Health Assistants

Picture this: you've got a health concern, but there's no need to book an appointment, wait for hours at the clinic, or rely on sporadic check-ups. Instead, a Virtual Health Assistant (VHA) is at your service 24/7, ready to offer advice, monitor your symptoms, and even schedule appointments if necessary. This isn't science fiction; it's the imminent reality in healthcare.

Virtual Health Assistants leverage the power of artificial intelligence to offer patients personalised health advice and support. These smart systems can process vast amounts of medical data, recognise patterns, and provide recommendations based on individual health profiles. Imagine a digital companion that knows your medical history, understands your current health status, and keeps track of your wellness goals. That's what VHAs promise to deliver.

One of the standout features of VHAs is their ability to engage patients continuously. This constant interaction can lead to better health outcomes by encouraging patients to take a proactive role in managing their health. Instead of being passive recipients of sporadic medical advice, patients become active participants in their healthcare journey. It's a bit like having a doctor in your pocket — although it doesn't come with a white coat and stethoscope.

Of course, VHAs aren't limited to just answering queries or reminding you to take your medication. Advanced systems are capable of conducting preliminary assessments based on symptoms you report. They can guide you through a series of questions to triage your condition, offering recommendations ranging from home remedies to suggesting you seek immediate medical attention if necessary. This can help alleviate the burden on healthcare professionals by filtering out less urgent cases.

Moreover, Virtual Health Assistants play a crucial role in chronic disease management. For patients living with conditions like diabetes, hypertension, or asthma, consistent monitoring and timely interventions are critical. VHAs can track vital signs, provide educational resources, and remind patients to adhere to their treatment plans. Think of them as the diligent, but slightly less annoying, version of a nagging parent.

Personalisation is another significant benefit of VHAs. These systems can learn from your interactions, adjusting the advice they provide based on your preferences and past responses. For example, if you're someone who responds better to positive reinforcement rather than strict admonitions, the VHA will adapt accordingly. There's no one-size-fits-all approach here; it's all about what works best for you.

However, it's not all sunshine and roses. The implementation of VHAs does raise several concerns, especially around data privacy and security. These systems need access to sensitive medical data to function effectively, which makes them potential targets for cyber-attacks. Ensuring that robust security measures are in place is paramount to gaining and maintaining patient trust. After all, no one wants their medical history to become a viral sensation on social media.

Alongside privacy concerns, there's also the question of accuracy. Medical advice, even from highly trained professionals, isn't infallible. Therefore, can we truly rely on an AI-driven assistant to provide accurate and safe health recommendations? The key here lies in the continuous improvement of these systems. As more data is collected and analysed, VHAs will become increasingly adept at offering reliable advice. But, like an apprentice chef, they'll need time and experience before we can fully trust their culinary—or in this case, medical—creations.

To enhance reliability, many developers of VHAs are integrating them with professional healthcare networks. This allows the systems to access up-to-date medical knowledge and guidelines, ensuring that the advice they provide is grounded in the latest evidence-based practices. Many VHAs also have built-in protocols to escalate cases that require human intervention, ensuring a safety net is always in place.

On the flip side, healthcare professionals stand to gain from the advent of VHAs. By automating routine tasks and preliminary assessments, these systems can free up valuable time for doctors and nurses to focus on more complex and urgent cases. This not only improves efficiency but also enhances job satisfaction and reduces burnout. So, while VHAs might not replace healthcare professionals, they could make their lives a whole lot easier.

Another intriguing aspect is the potential for VHAs to democratise access to healthcare. In regions where medical services are scarce or overloaded, having a virtual assistant can bridge the gap. It can offer basic healthcare advice and monitor patients remotely, making it a valuable tool in rural and underserved areas. It's the digital equivalent of bringing healthcare to your doorstep, only without the muddy boots.

The journey towards widespread adoption of VHAs won't be without its bumps and scrapes. Regulatory hurdles, technological challenges, and the need for public buy-in are all part of the landscape. But as we've seen with other technological advancements, persistence and innovation often pave the way for acceptance and integration.

In conclusion, Virtual Health Assistants hold immense promise for enhancing patient engagement in healthcare. They offer a personalised, continuous, and proactive approach to healthcare management, empowering patients and healthcare professionals alike. While there are legitimate concerns around privacy, accuracy, and acceptance, the potential benefits make it a sector worth watching. As these digital companions become more sophisticated and integrated into our healthcare systems, they may very well become an indispensable part of our wellness journey.

As the healthcare sector grapples with increasing demands and limited resources, VHAs represent an exciting frontier in delivering better care to more people. And who knows? In a few years, chatting with your virtual health assistant might become as commonplace as checking your email or streaming your favourite TV series. The future, it seems, is not just virtual; it's also healthy.

Chatbots and Virtual Consultations have heralded a new era in the patient care continuum, blending cutting-edge AI technology with everyday healthcare interactions. It's not just about convenience—for some, it can be a game-changer, offering medical advice round the clock without needing a face-to-face doctor's appointment.

For patients, navigating the complex rhythms of their health can often feel like deciphering an enigma wrapped in labyrinthine medical jargon. Enter the chatbot, a digital Florence Nightingale ready to provide instant responses, reminders, and care tips, all at one's fingertips. Whether it's a late-night query about a rash or understanding the side effects of a new medication, chatbots have the uncanny ability to provide immediate assistance.

Take, for example, the virtual health assistant, a subset of chatbots designed to perform tasks beyond mere Q&A. These digital assistants delve deeper into patient records, offering tailored medical advice. They can cross-reference symptoms with historical data, much like a seasoned practitioner might, and alert patients about medication schedules or upcoming appointments. A chatbot's ability to triage based on symptomatology could even drastically alleviate the burden on emergency services, directing non-urgent cases to appropriate alternatives.

However, let's not get too starry-eyed. While these bots can handle a myriad of tasks, they aren't foolproof. The possibility of misinterpretation looms, especially when patients describe symptoms ambiguously. Despite these limitations, the fact remains that chatbots proffer a layer of accessibility that traditional models of healthcare struggle to match. This added layer is crucial, particularly in underserved communities where medical resources are scarce.

What about virtual consultations? These are essentially video calls with medical professionals, facilitated through sophisticated algorithms that help in diagnosis and management. Imagine a world where you could consult a healthcare specialist from the comfort of your home, saving time and resources on commutes and hospital wait times. It's perhaps one of the most poignant demonstrations of how AI can bring about patient-centric care.

The reach of virtual consultations is profound. They bridge geographical disparate gaps, bringing expert healthcare to remote areas. Picture rural localities where medical facilities are few and far between. Virtual consultations can democratise healthcare access, offering those living in seclusion the chance to receive specialist care without the logistical nightmare of traveling to a big city.

From a financial perspective, virtual consultations are proving to be cost-effective for healthcare systems worldwide. Think of the operational costs saved—from hospital maintenance to manpower allocation. Not to say these consultations completely eliminate the need for hospital visits, but they certainly act as a preliminary line of defence, filtering those who genuinely need in-person medical interventions from those who can be managed remotely.

Now, if you're wondering about the human touch, fret not. Virtual consultations are designed to augment, not replace, the human element in healthcare. In this digital handshake, patients often report a sense of empathy and personal care, contrary to the cold, mechanical interaction some might expect. Many virtual platforms even incorporate biometric readings and environmental sensing to create a more holistic diagnostic process.

Behind the scenes, the integration of natural language processing (NLP) and machine learning ensures these consultations are as close to a real-world experience as possible. Algorithms constantly learn from ongoing interactions, refining their accuracy and the quality of care over time. They might even flag anomalies missed by overworked, stressed human eyes, adding an extra layer of scrutiny to patient care.

In conclusion, chatbots and virtual consultations manifest the seismic shifts AI is channeling into the healthcare sector. They offer not just a glimpse but a firm footing into what the future might hold—where immediacy, accessibility, and personalized care converge to ensure a more efficient, equitable, and patient-centered healthcare system.

Wearable Technology and Remote Monitoring

Wearable technology and remote monitoring are revolutionising the way we approach patient engagement. These innovations are no longer the stuff of sci-fi dreams but are readily available and increasingly integrated into our daily lives. The healthcare industry has been quick to adopt these technologies, and for good reason. Wearable devices, from smartwatches to more specialised medical equipment, enable continuous health monitoring, providing real-time data that is crucial for both patients and healthcare providers.

The beauty of wearable technology lies in its ability to collect a plethora of data points without being intrusive. From tracking heart rates and sleep patterns to measuring blood glucose levels and monitoring physical activity, these devices cover a wide range of health metrics. This data isn't just stored and forgotten; it can be transmitted to healthcare providers, enabling more informed and timely medical decisions. The implications for patient engagement are significant. Patients are not just passive recipients of care; they're active participants, armed with data about their health.

The Gen Z crowd might treat their smartwatches as mere fitness gadgets, but for elderly patients or those with chronic conditions, these devices can be life-changing. Remote monitoring technology allows for continuous oversight of critical health indicators, drastically reducing the need for frequent hospital visits. Imagine a diabetic patient who no longer needs to prick their finger daily because their glucose levels are constantly monitored by a device that sends alerts to both the patient and their doctor. It's like living with a virtual healthcare assistant strapped to your wrist.

It's not all rainbows and butterflies, though. There are considerable challenges to widespread adoption, ranging from data privacy concerns to the accuracy of the measurements taken by these devices. Let's face it, no one wants their health data hacked or shared without their consent. Wearable tech companies are under intense scrutiny to ensure that the data security protocols they employ are rock solid. Moreover, there's also the question of regulatory approval. The medical field isn't quite as lenient as the tech world when it comes to new innovations. A device that counts your steps might fly under the radar, but one that promises to diagnose heart conditions had better be as reliable as the ECG machine in your doctor's office.

Yet, despite these challenges, the potential benefits far outweigh the drawbacks. Consider the role of remote monitoring in managing chronic diseases. Conditions like hypertension, diabetes, and chronic obstructive pulmonary disease (COPD) require ongoing management and can lead to severe complications if not carefully monitored. Wearable technology enables constant vigilance, making it easier to keep these conditions in check. This constant stream of data allows for a level of precision in treatment plans that was previously unimaginable.

But wait, there's more. Wearable technology can also play a critical role in preventive healthcare. It's not just about managing existing conditions but about preventing them from emerging in the first place. Take cardiovascular health, for example. Early detection of irregularities through continuous heart rate monitoring can prompt timely interventions, potentially preventing serious conditions like strokes or heart attacks. Similarly, tracking physical activity and encouraging a more active lifestyle can go a long way in preventing diseases associated with sedentary behaviour.

Furthermore, the integration of wearable technology with AI and machine learning algorithms opens up new avenues for healthcare innovations. These algorithms can analyse the massive amounts of data generated by wearable devices to identify trends and make predictive analyses. For instance, an AI-powered system can predict potential health issues and flag them for both patients and healthcare providers. This combination moves us from descriptive to prescriptive healthcare, offering proactive solutions instead of reactive treatments.

What about the role of behavioural economics in all of this? Incentivising patients to use wearable technology regularly can be a game-changer. Insurance companies are already jumping on this bandwagon, offering discounts or rewards for policyholders who actively use wearables to monitor their health metrics. This approach not only promotes healthier lifestyles but also reduces healthcare costs in the long run. It's a win-win scenario: patients stay healthier, and insurance companies save money.

One can't ignore the social implications either. Wearable technology can bridge the gap between healthcare professionals and patients, especially in underserved or remote areas. Not everyone has easy access to top-notch medical facilities, but nearly everyone has access to technology. Telemedicine, empowered by data from wearable devices, can enable healthcare providers to offer consultations and medical advice to people living in far-flung areas. This democratisation of healthcare is one of the most exciting promises of wearable technology and remote monitoring.

The narrative wouldn't be complete without mentioning the mental health aspect. Wearables that track physiological metrics can also provide insights into mental well-being. Features that monitor stress levels, sleep quality and even activity reminders can have a tangible impact on mental health management. Stress and mental health issues are notoriously hard to quantify, but continuous monitoring provides invaluable data, helping healthcare providers to offer more personalised treatments.

The future looks promising, but let's not pop the champagne just yet. Many of these technologies are still in their infancy, and there's much work to be done in terms of research, validation, and regulatory approval. Collaborative efforts between tech companies, healthcare providers, and regulatory bodies will be key to overcoming these hurdles. Ensuring equitable access to these technologies is another concern that needs to be addressed. While the tech-savvy urban population might be quick to adopt these changes, ensuring that rural and less affluent populations aren't left behind will be crucial.

In summary, wearable technology and remote monitoring have the potential to drastically improve patient engagement and overall healthcare outcomes. From managing chronic conditions to preventing new ones, these innovations offer a multifaceted approach to healthcare. However, significant challenges remain, particularly in the realms of data security, accuracy, and regulatory approval. As these issues are addressed, the widespread adoption of wearable technology promises to revolutionise the healthcare landscape, making it more engaging, proactive, and inclusive.

Chapter 7:
Ethical and Legal Considerations

As AI meanders its way into healthcare, the ethical and legal implications seem to be multiplying faster than algorithms can compute. Data privacy, a term we once whispered about in hushed tones, now screams for our attention. While the allure of machine-assisted diagnoses and bespoke treatment plans wows, we can't gloss over the stark realities of decision-making and accountability. What happens when a machine errs? And will bureaucrats race the algorithms to set the guardrails before the next big data breach? The juxtaposition of innovation and regulation conjures up a fascinatingly fraught dialogue, leaving us to ponder not just what AI can do for healthcare, but also what it ethically should do.

Data Privacy and Security

When you're dealing with healthcare, data privacy and security can't be taken lightly. These two elements form the cornerstone of ethical AI deployment in medical settings. Imagine a world where your medical records, a trove of deeply personal information, are up for grabs due to lax security measures. The consequences aren't just limited to individual privacy breaches; they can escalate into a public health crisis if sensitive information falls into the wrong hands.

One of the key issues is the sheer volume and sensitivity of healthcare data. Health records contain everything from your medical history to details about your genetic makeup. In the context of AI, this data needs to be stored, processed, and analysed at scales never seen before. This vast amount of information creates numerous entry points for potential breaches, making robust data security protocols an absolute necessity. But maintaining these protocols isn't as simple as flicking a switch; it requires ongoing vigilance and continual adaptation to newer threats.

Let's not forget that healthcare data is an attractive target for cybercriminals. Unlike financial data, you can't simply cancel a health record. If compromised, the consequences can be long-lasting, affecting everything from your employability to your insurability. This makes the healthcare sector uniquely vulnerable and necessitates top-notch security measures.

Moreover, there's the matter of compliance with various legal frameworks. In the UK, you have the Data Protection Act 2018 which aligns with the EU's General Data Protection Regulation (GDPR). These laws are designed to protect individuals' privacy and provide a regulatory framework for the use of personal data. Failing to comply with these regulations can not only result in hefty fines but also erode public trust, which is paramount when it comes to healthcare.

But it's not just about throwing a firewall around your data and calling it a day. Authentication protocols have to be rock-solid. Two-factor authentication is almost a must-have in today's environment. Role-based access controls (RBAC) are another vital aspect. Not everyone needs access to all information, and restricting data access based on job roles can significantly mitigate risks.

Encryption plays a vital role here. Data must be encrypted, both at rest and in transit, to ensure that even if it does fall into the wrong hands, it is rendered useless. Modern encryption methods are robust, but they require continuous updates to stay ahead of emerging threats. It's a cat-and-mouse game where the stakes are incredibly high.

The ethical implications of data privacy go beyond just compliance and security measures. There's a moral obligation to consider how data is used. Informed consent is a critical facet here. Patients need to be informed about what data is being collected, how it will be used, and who will have access to it. Moreover, they should have the option to opt out without facing repercussions in their treatment.

Also worth noting is the potential for bias in AI algorithms. If the data fed into the AI is biased, the outcomes will be too. This can perpetuate existing inequalities in the healthcare system. Careful auditing and continual monitoring of AI algorithms are necessary to ensure that they are both fair and equitable.

Incorporating blockchain technology offers another layer of security and transparency. While still an emerging field, blockchain could provide immutable records that are tamper-evident. This technology ensures that once data is written, it can't be changed, thus providing a trustworthy log of who accessed what and when.

You also can't ignore the importance of incident response plans. Given the complexity and sophistication of modern cyber-attacks, even the most secure systems can be breached. Having a quick, effective response plan can mitigate the damage caused by such incidents. Regular drills and updates to the response plan are essential components of a holistic security strategy.

Furthermore, engaging with third-party vendors introduces another layer of complexity. Your data security is only as strong as the weakest link in the chain. It is crucial to conduct thorough due diligence and regular audits of any third parties involved in handling healthcare data. Contracts should clearly outline data protection responsibilities and provide for penalties in case of non-compliance.

AI systems must also support data anonymisation techniques. This involves stripping data of identifiable information to protect patient privacy while still allowing for meaningful analysis. It's a balancing act between data utility and privacy, but one that's necessary as we navigate this brave new world.

Finally, continuous education and training for healthcare professionals on data security best practices can't be overstated. Human error is often a significant vulnerability, whether it's through phishing attacks, mishandling data, or simply negligence. Regular training sessions and updates on emerging threats can significantly reduce these risks.

And let's not forget the public's role in this. Educated patients are more likely to understand the importance of data security and privacy, and they'll be more willing to participate in AI-driven healthcare initiatives. Transparency about how data is used and protected can go a long way in building this trust.

In conclusion, the integration of AI in healthcare presents an unprecedented opportunity to improve patient outcomes and streamline operations. However, with these advancements come heightened risks to data privacy and security. Implementing strong technical safeguards, ensuring legal compliance, fostering a culture of ethical data usage, and maintaining patient trust are critical components that must not be overlooked. The road ahead is fraught with challenges, but with careful consideration and proactive measures, the benefits far outweigh the risks.

Decision-Making and Accountability

As we dive into the integration of AI within the healthcare sector, it's crucial to examine how decision-making and accountability are evolving. AI can process vast amounts of data quickly, making it a powerful tool for diagnosing diseases, personalising treatments, and managing hospital operations. However, the increased reliance on AI raises pressing ethical and legal questions about responsibility and transparency.

One critical concern is who should be held accountable when an AI system makes an error. In a traditional medical setting, the onus falls on the healthcare provider. With AI, it's less clear. If an AI system misdiagnoses a patient, is the blame to be laid at the feet of the software developers, the healthcare providers, or even the health institutions that deploy these systems? The lines blur, making it essential to establish clear frameworks for responsibility.

Typically, AI systems are designed to support, not replace, human decision-making. However, as these systems become more sophisticated, the boundary between support and replacement starts to fade. For instance, predictive analytics can offer early detection of diseases, but they also raise questions about how much trust physicians should place in these predictions. When AI can potentially outperform humans in diagnostic accuracy, the stakes in decision-making grow exponentially.

On the other hand, we must consider the ethical implications of automated decision-making in healthcare. Algorithms can inadvertently introduce biases based on the data they're trained on. If an AI system has been trained predominantly on data from one demographic group, its recommendations might not be applicable to other groups. This potential for bias necessitates rigorous validation and continuous monitoring of AI systems to ensure equitable healthcare.

Moreover, the opacity—or the "black box" nature—of many AI models complicates decision-making. Machine learning algorithms, especially deep learning models, can be incredibly complex, making it difficult to understand how they derive their conclusions. This lack of transparency can be problematic for healthcare professionals who need to interpret these results and for patients who deserve to know how decisions about their health are being made.

Implementing AI in healthcare also requires a shift in how professionals are trained to think about and interact with these systems. It's not just about understanding how to use the tools but also about developing a critical mindset to question and validate AI recommendations. Medical curriculums will need to incorporate training in AI literacy to prepare future healthcare providers. This ongoing education is vital for making informed decisions and holding parties accountable.

From a legal perspective, the questions of liability become even murkier. Current regulations are struggling to keep pace with technological advancements. Policymakers must update legal frameworks to account for AI's role in healthcare. These new regulations should address the accountability of healthcare providers, technology companies, and even the AI systems themselves. The challenge is to create laws that are robust enough to protect patients while not stifling innovation.

Interestingly, some suggest the concept of "explainable AI" as a solution to the transparency issue. Explainable AI aims to make the reasoning behind AI decisions more understandable to humans. If an AI system can explain its decision-making process in a way that healthcare providers can grasp, it becomes easier to audit these decisions and hold the appropriate party accountable. However, achieving this level of explainability without sacrificing performance is a significant technical challenge.

Additionally, informed consent takes on a new dimension in the age of AI. Patients need to be made aware when AI systems are being used in their diagnosis or treatment. They should also understand the potential benefits and risks associated with these technologies. This calls for developing new consent protocols that can effectively communicate these complexities to patients.

Data governance is another important factor. AI systems rely heavily on data, and the quality of this data can significantly impact their performance. Establishing robust data governance frameworks ensures that the data used is accurate, representative, and ethically sourced. Clear guidelines on data ownership, access, and usage are imperative for maintaining accountability. Such regulations should also address the scenarios in which data needs to be shared across different healthcare providers and stakeholders.

Medical ethics often operates on the principle of "do no harm". As AI begins to play a pivotal role in healthcare decision-making, this principle must extend to the design and deployment of these systems. Developers and healthcare providers must engage in thorough testing and validation processes to minimise risks of harm. Ethical oversight committees might be necessary to review AI systems and their applications in healthcare settings.

Public trust in AI will largely hinge on how well these systems can demonstrate accountability and ethical integrity. Transparency about system limitations and potential risks is crucial. When errors occur, a transparent process for analysing what went wrong and implementing corrective actions can build public trust. Moreover, involving diverse stakeholders in the development and implementation of AI systems can help address various ethical concerns and ensure more balanced decision-making.

One forward-thinking approach is the concept of "human-in-the-loop" AI, where human oversight is built into the AI decision-making process. This hybrid model can combine the strengths of human intuition and judgment with the computational power of AI. For example, an AI system might flag potential health problems, but a human doctor would review these flags before making final decisions.

This method helps distribute responsibility and ensures that AI remains a tool rather than the final arbiter.

Ultimately, the integration of AI in healthcare is not just a technological shift; it's a cultural and ethical one as well. Decision-making frameworks will need to adapt, and roles within healthcare may need redefinition. Developing a comprehensive approach to accountability will require collaboration among technologists, healthcare providers, ethicists, and legal experts. Only through such multi-faceted efforts can we ensure that AI in healthcare serves its intended purpose—advancing medical science and improving patient outcomes—while upholding the highest standards of ethical accountability.

As with any transformative technology, the road ahead is riddled with challenges, but it's also filled with opportunities for improving healthcare delivery. By taking a proactive stance on decision-making and accountability, we can navigate these complexities and harness the full potential of AI to revolutionise healthcare for the better.

Chapter 8:
Training and Education for
Healthcare Professionals

As the healthcare sector grapples with the rapid infusion of artificial intelligence (AI), training and education for healthcare professionals have taken on unprecedented urgency. Today's doctors, nurses, and allied health workers can no longer coast on traditional methods; they must be adept at navigating the digital landscape. Integrating AI into medical curriculums is no longer a futuristic concept but a practical necessity. Medical schools and training programs are adapting, albeit at varied paces, with some institutions leading the charge in teaching the next generation of healthcare professionals to utilise AI tools effectively. Continuous learning and adaptation are paramount, as the technology landscape shifts faster than a seasoned consultant's schedule. The challenge lies not only in teaching the theoretical aspects but also in fostering a culture that embraces continuous professional development and the willingness to evolve with technological advancements. This paradigm shift is essential for preparing healthcare workers to harness AI's full potential and improve patient care outcomes substantially.

Integrating AI into Medical Curriculums

It's clear that the incorporation of artificial intelligence (AI) into healthcare isn't just a fleeting trend—it's a seismic shift that will fundamentally reshape how we approach medicine. But here's the kicker: none of this transformative potential can be realised if our healthcare professionals aren't prepared. That's where integrating AI into medical curriculums comes in.

Training the next generation of doctors, nurses, and healthcare workers to navigate a world replete with AI technologies demands thorough and thoughtful changes in medical education. Medical schools currently focus heavily on core biological sciences, clinical skills, and patient interactions. However, the future curriculum must also embrace IT literacy, data analytics, and the ethical implications of AI in healthcare. This is not just an add-on but a necessity.

Consider the role of AI in diagnostics. Machine learning algorithms can now analyse images and detect conditions like cancer or fractures more rapidly and, in some cases, more accurately than human doctors. These advancements should be a central focus in radiology courses. Students should work on case studies where AI applications are used, understand their limitations, and learn how to interpret AI-generated results. Additionally, simulations incorporating AI diagnosing tools can offer hands-on experience before even stepping into a hospital.

A balanced curriculum should integrate AI education with core medical subjects without overwhelming the students. One approach might be to implement interdisciplinary courses that combine elements of data science and medicine. Such courses could explore how AI models are built and validated, giving future doctors a robust understanding of the tools they'll be using.

A potential pitfall is the "black box" nature of AI, where the decision-making process of algorithms can be opaque even to their creators. Medical curriculums need to address this head-on by fostering critical thinking skills. Apart from learning how to use AI tools, healthcare professionals must ask pertinent questions about the data being fed into these systems and the science behind the algorithms' decisions. This cultivates a dual expertise: one part rooted in technical know-how, the other in rigorous medical ethics.

There's also the ethical dimension, a topic not just relevant but crucial. AI will make consequential decisions, sometimes autonomously. So, medical ethics education must now cover new ground. Concepts like bias in AI, accountability for AI-driven decisions, and ensuring equitable access to AI technology should become standard parts of the medical ethics curriculum. If AI is the scalpel of the 21st century, its ethical use is the steady hand.

Additionally, partnerships between medical schools and tech companies can be instrumental. Collaboration can ensure that the curriculum remains up-to-date with the latest technological developments. Medical students can benefit from internships and research opportunities at tech firms specialising in healthcare AI. Such real-world experiences will deepen their understanding and prepare them for practical challenges.

Historically, medical education has been slow to adapt to new technology, but integrating AI into curriculums can't afford the luxury of time. The fast-paced evolution of technology necessitates an equally agile educational framework. Medical institutions should partner with AI experts to continuously revise and update their courses. Continuous feedback loops can help ensure that what's taught is what's needed in practice.

We also shouldn't forget the importance of teaching faculty. Many current medical educators may lack the expertise to teach AI-focused subjects. This is an area that will require investment, both in terms of hiring new faculty members who specialise in AI and retraining existing staff. Workshops, seminars, and short courses can help existing educators get up to speed. After all, it's one thing to overhaul a curriculum on paper, and another entirely to deliver it effectively.

The bureaucratic hurdles in academia can make rapid changes challenging, but ensuring our next generation of healthcare professionals is well-versed in AI is a challenge worth taking on. Medical accreditation bodies should be ready to adapt and evolve their standards. They must recognise the importance of AI and ensure medical schools across the nation align their curriculums accordingly. The early adopters will set the benchmark for others to follow.

Healthcare professionals are lifelong learners by the very nature of their calling, and the medical curriculum should serve as the first mile in an endless marathon of learning. Early exposure to AI can inspire curiosity and self-directed learning. Students who have already seen the potential of AI in their studies will be more likely to engage in continuous professional development courses and certifications related to AI throughout their careers.

A significant element involves integrating AI into the practical aspects of medical training. Just as simulations play a pivotal role in traditional medical training, AI-driven simulations can recreate complex clinical scenarios that require quick decision-making. Virtual patients, equipped with AI algorithms to simulate real-world variability, can be invaluable educational tools. These virtual encounters offer low-stakes environments for students to practice diagnosing, planning treatments, and making complex decisions.

Moreover, the future of clinical rotations may include substantial use of AI. Imagine students rotating through departments where AI is actively utilised in diagnostics, patient monitoring, and even treatment decisions. Such exposure will help them not only understand AI's capabilities but also see firsthand how it integrates into the day-to-day workflow of healthcare providers.

Let's also not overlook the softer skills. Communication, teamwork, and adaptability are paramount. AI might revolutionise medicine, but it won't replace the human touch. Hence, medical curriculums must stress that AI is a tool to augment healthcare, not replace the crucial human elements. Courses that teach students to collaborate with AI and use it as a supplement to their skills will be invaluable.

Moreover, the ongoing relationship between healthcare professionals and AI will be symbiotic. AI has the capacity to learn and improve constantly, offering up-to-date information spanning vast medical literature repositories, something no single human can achieve. In return, healthcare professionals who understand the inner workings of AI can provide key insights to improve these systems further. Medical curriculums should highlight this dynamic, preparing students not only to use AI but to contribute to its evolution.

In summary, integrating AI into medical curriculums is an absolute necessity if we're to leverage the full potential of this technology in transforming healthcare. This revolution isn't just coming—it's here. The complexity of medicine demands that we prepare our future healthcare professionals to harness the power of AI while respecting the ethical, clinical, and human aspects of their work. Anything less would be a failure to seize one of the most promising advancements in medical history.

Continuous Learning and Adaptation

Let's face it: the healthcare world is not what it used to be. Gone are the days of static medical knowledge that doctors could tuck away in their heads forever. Instead, the pace of change is dizzying, and this couldn't be truer than with AI's foray into healthcare. The evolution of AI technologies requires that healthcare professionals remain constantly engaged in learning and adapting. It's not just about staying updated—it's about thriving in an ever-changing landscape.

Creating a "continuous learning culture" is no longer optional for healthcare institutions. It's a sheer necessity. AI algorithms grow smarter, electronic health records become more integrated, and predictive analytics improve daily. The knowledge gained five years ago might already be outdated or even irrelevant. Professional development must thus shift from sporadic training sessions to an ongoing process of improvement and adaptation.

The approach to continuous learning needs to be holistic. It's not solely about attending workshops or earning Continuing Medical Education (CME) credits. Practitioners have to familiarize themselves with the latest tools, understand new algorithms, and comprehend the ethical implications of data-driven decisions. This might sound like juggling ten plates simultaneously, but the consequences of failing to adapt are far too severe—from misguided treatment plans to potential breaches in patient confidentiality.

Healthcare organizations should invest heavily in training programs that evolve in concert with technological advancements. Just as AI and machine learning are dynamic, so too must be the programs designed to educate healthcare professionals. Online courses, interactive modules, VR simulations, and hands-on workshops can bridge the gap between traditional education and the new, tech-infused reality healthcare workers face. The aim should be to create a seamless blend of theoretical knowledge and practical application.

But, of course, change brings challenges. One significant barrier to continuous learning is the "learning curve" itself, which can seem daunting. Many healthcare professionals, particularly those who've been practising for decades, may feel overwhelmed or resistant to adopting new technologies. There's also the practical issue of time—how do busy practitioners find the hours needed to update their skills?

To mitigate these issues, training programs should be adaptive and personalised, much like the AI solutions they aim to teach. Tailored learning experiences that reflect an individual healthcare professional's prior knowledge and specific needs can make continuous education less of a chore and more of an engaging process. Micro-learning modules can offer flexibility, allowing professionals to learn at their own pace and in manageable segments.

The role of collaboration cannot be overstated. Often, the best learning happens through interaction with colleagues and constant immersion in communal knowledge. Hospitals and clinics can foster environments that encourage knowledge sharing, perhaps by setting up "innovation hubs" where multidisciplinary teams work together on real-world problems, using the latest AI tools and methodologies. These collaborations can serve as live case studies from which everyone can learn and adapt.

Professional societies and medical boards also have crucial parts to play. They must update accreditation standards to include competencies in AI and data analytics. Offering incentives for continual professional development, perhaps through recognition programs or even requirement mandates, could push more healthcare workers into perpetual education mode. Beyond institutions, there's a social responsibility angle too—ensuring that the public remains confident in healthcare services, knowing that practitioners are well-versed in the latest advancements.

Critically, continuous learning isn't about technology alone. It's about understanding patient interactions in an AI-enhanced world. As AI tools help diagnose diseases or suggest treatment plans, healthcare professionals need to balance these recommendations with the human touch. Learning how to communicate effectively about AI-driven decisions and maintaining empathy is an equally important, albeit often overlooked, aspect of ongoing education.

Moreover, the world of AI and technology comes with its set of ethical quandaries. Professionals must stay updated on these evolving discussions—whether it's about bias in algorithms or the scope of data use. Ethical training should be integrated into continuous education to prepare professionals for the complex decision-making processes that lie ahead.

Ultimately, continuous learning and adaptation aren't end goals but ongoing journeys. As AI continues to revolutionise the healthcare sector, professionals must commit to a lifelong learning mindset. No one's suggesting it's going to be easy. However, the potential rewards—a better quality of care, more accurate diagnoses, and heightened efficiency—make the effort undeniably worth it.

Chapter 9:
AI in Public Health

In this chapter, we'll take a closer look at how artificial intelligence is set to revolutionise public health like never before. Picture this: algorithms sifting through mountains of data to predict and manage epidemics before they spiral out of control. It's as if AI has become the Sherlock Holmes of the healthcare world, only quicker and without the nicotine addiction. Beyond epidemic tracking, AI's prowess in population health analytics allows for a more nuanced understanding of health trends and resource allocation. With AI-driven insights, public health policies could become sharper than ever, targeting problems with surgical precision. In essence, the fusion of AI and public health isn't just a fancy upgrade; it's a paradigm shift poised to redefine how we approach communal well-being. Whether it's crunching numbers or spotting an anomaly in health data, the AI systems of the near future promise to make public health monitoring almost art-like in its complexity and efficacy.

Tracking and Managing Epidemics

Until recently, epidemic tracking has largely relied on traditional methodologies—gathering data from hospitals, clinics, and laboratories, then painstakingly analysing it to detect trends and outbreaks. This is a cumbersome, often delayed process that can cost precious time in preventing the spread of infectious diseases. But, in an age where AI is revolutionising nearly every sector, public health hasn't been left behind.

Artificial Intelligence is proving to be a game-changer in the realm of epidemic tracking and management. By harnessing the power of machine learning algorithms and big data analytics, health officials can now track the spread of diseases in real-time, giving them an invaluable head start in deploying treatments and preventive measures. Think of it as the difference between using a vintage map and a real-time GPS; the former might get you to your destination eventually, but the latter ensures you get there swiftly and accurately.

Consider the myriad sources from which AI systems draw their data: social media activity, search engine queries, healthcare records, and even wearable health technology. By analysing this vast amount of information, AI can identify outbreaks at their nascent stages, long before they would traditionally be detected. For example, search terms such as "flu symptoms" can spike in a particular geographic area, alerting public health authorities even before patients start filling up waiting rooms.

Taking it a step further, AI can model potential scenarios for epidemic spread, allowing for predictive analytics that help in planning and resource allocation. Such models can consider countless variables, including population density, travel patterns, and even weather conditions, to forecast where and how quickly a disease might spread. This is not science fiction; it's happening right now. During the COVID-19 pandemic, AI-driven models were instrumental in predicting hotspots, which allowed for more focused lockdowns and resource distribution.

In addition to forecasting, AI also has a role in real-time management. As an epidemic unfolds, the situation can change by the hour. AI systems can continuously analyse new data and revise their predictions and recommendations accordingly. This dynamic reactivity is something human analysts, no matter how skilled, simply can't match.

But let's not get too carried away with the possibilities. AI is not a silver bullet. It requires data, and lots of it, which must be clean, accurate, and timely. This presents its own set of challenges, especially in regions where healthcare infrastructure is lacking. There are also concerns around privacy and the ethical use of data, particularly when utilising personal health information from wearables and social media.

However, the potential benefits are undeniable. For example, in the fight against antibiotic resistance—a growing global threat—AI can identify patterns in prescription and infection rates far quicker than traditional methods. This allows for more targeted public health interventions, potentially saving thousands of lives and billions in healthcare costs.

The technology also shines in developing treatment protocols during an epidemic. AI can analyse the effectiveness of different treatment methods in real-time, suggesting the best course of action based on continually updated data. This is particularly useful in scenarios where a novel pathogen is involved, and time is of the essence.

Let's not ignore the role of AI in vaccine development either. The traditional timeline for developing a vaccine can span years. With AI, we can potentially reduce this to months. By analysing genetic data and simulating various biological scenarios, AI can identify likely candidates for vaccine development far quicker than conventional methods. This was evident during the COVID-19 pandemic when AI algorithms helped researchers understand the virus's structure and behaviour much faster than in any previous viral outbreak.

Moreover, AI can aid in the logistical challenges that come with managing an epidemic. From optimising the distribution of medical supplies to ensuring healthcare facilities are not overwhelmed, AI's capabilities extend beyond mere data analysis. For instance, during the peak of the COVID-19 pandemic, AI systems were used to manage

ICU capacities and ventilator distributions, ensuring that resources were allocated efficiently and equitably.

As promising as AI is, it's crucial to note the importance of human oversight. AI provides the tools and insights, but decisions ultimately rest with public health officials and medical professionals. AI's role is akin to that of an astute advisor—offering insights, predictions, and recommendations—but it is the humans who must interpret and act upon this information wisely. Effective epidemic management will always require this symbiosis between human intuition and AI-driven analytics.

We must also consider the global implications. Epidemics don't respect borders, and neither should our countermeasures. There's potential for a global AI-driven network for tracking and managing epidemics—one that shares data, models, and strategies. This kind of international cooperation could revolutionize how we handle global health crises, making it possible to snuff out the embers of an outbreak before they become an uncontrollable blaze.

But the road ahead isn't without its bumps. Integrating AI into public health systems requires not just technological advancements but also significant policy and infrastructural changes. Public health authorities will need to invest not only in AI tools but also in training personnel to use these tools effectively. There will be challenges around data sharing, both within and between countries, and questions about who controls, accesses, and benefits from this data.

Yet, despite these challenges, the promise of AI in tracking and managing epidemics is too significant to ignore. The combination of rapid data analysis, predictive modelling, and real-time management capabilities presents a potent arsenal against future public health threats. As we continue to refine these technologies and address the ethical, logistical, and infrastructural hurdles, we edge closer to a world where the devastation wrought by epidemics and pandemics can be significantly mitigated.

In conclusion, while AI won't eliminate the threat of epidemics, it offers new and powerful ways to track, manage, and ultimately contain them. In the ever-evolving landscape of public health, AI is not just a tool but a vital ally in the ongoing battle against infectious diseases. Whether it's through detecting outbreaks before they spread widely, optimizing resource allocation, or accelerating vaccine development, AI is poised to transform our approach to public health fundamentally. The future may still hold uncertainties, but one thing seems clear: in the war against epidemics, AI is a force to be reckoned with.

Population Health Analytics

In a world where data is the new oil, it's no surprise that public health is tapping into the power of analytics. Population health analytics, driven by artificial intelligence, is revolutionising how we manage public health. It's reshaping how we think about disease prevention, health promotion, and even policy-making.

The primary objective of population health analytics is to aggregate and analyse health data from various sources. These sources range from electronic health records to social determinants of health, including environmental data, demographic information, and even socioeconomic factors. By doing so, AI enables public health professionals to identify trends and patterns that were previously invisible in the sea of data. The big idea? To anticipate health outcomes and to intervene before problems escalate.

One key application is predictive modelling. By analysing historical data, AI can predict future outbreaks of diseases or health issues within specific communities. For instance, predictive models can forecast the likelihood of flu outbreaks by examining past flu seasons' data, current meteorological conditions, and social media activity. Sounds futuristic? Well, it's already happening. This level of foresight enables health officials to allocate resources more efficiently and implement targeted interventions well in advance.

Moreover, AI's ability to cross-reference and analyse vast datasets makes it invaluable in identifying health disparities across different populations. This can shine a light on segments of the population that may be at risk of specific health issues due to socio-economic factors, geographic locations, or genetic predispositions. If we can identify these inequalities, we can channel resources and health initiatives where they are most needed, promoting equity in healthcare.

Beyond prediction, population health analytics also supports real-time monitoring. With AI systems in place, health departments can constantly monitor a wide array of data sources. This real-time surveillance can detect aberrations: sudden spikes in disease incidence, unusual patterns of symptoms, or even unexpected medication use. When an anomaly is flagged, it allows for rapid response, potentially averting a full-blown health crisis.

An innovative example of such real-time monitoring is the use of AI in tracking epidemic spread. Think back to the Zika virus or the more recent COVID-19 pandemic; how different would our response have been if we had AI-driven models monitoring and predicting the virus's spread in real-time? It's not just about having the data but having the means to process and interpret it instantaneously.

Another powerful tool in population health analytics is natural language processing (NLP). This AI technology can sift through vast amounts of unstructured data, such as clinical notes or social media posts. By extracting relevant information, NLP can contribute to understanding health trends and making timely decisions. Imagine the potential for early detection of mental health crises from social media activity or analysing massive amounts of patient feedback to identify common issues in healthcare delivery.

As if that weren't enough, AI can also enhance the efficacy of public health campaigns. By analysing data on demographic behaviour, AI can help tailor public health messages to resonate with different segments of the population. For instance, a public health campaign designed to encourage vaccination can be fine-tuned to address specific concerns or misconceptions prevalent in various communities. Effective communication can lead to higher engagement and better health outcomes, making the whole campaign more successful.

However, it's not all sunshine and roses. The use of AI in population health analytics brings to the forefront numerous ethical and legal considerations. Data privacy is a significant concern, as the more data you collect, the greater the risk of potential breaches. There's also the issue of data security, given that health data is particularly sensitive and often targeted by cybercriminals. Balancing the need for comprehensive data collection and respecting individual privacy is a tightrope walk that requires careful consideration and robust legal frameworks.

Additionally, there's the matter of algorithmic bias. If the data used to train AI models is not representative of the entire population, the predictions and insights generated could be skewed. This can inadvertently exacerbate health disparities rather than alleviate them. Transparency in AI algorithms and continuous monitoring for bias are imperative to ensure fair outcomes for all sections of the population. In a system designed to serve the greater good, bias can have devastating consequences; hence, it needs to be meticulously managed.

The integration of AI into population health analytics also necessitates an overhaul of skills among public health professionals. There's a growing need for expertise in data science, machine learning, and AI. This calls for new training programs and educational initiatives to equip the public health workforce with the necessary skills. After all, AI is a tool, and like any tool, its effectiveness hinges on how well it's used by those who wield it.

Cross-sector collaboration plays a crucial role too. Population health analytics isn't solely the responsibility of public health departments. It involves a myriad of partners, including healthcare providers, academic institutions, technology companies, and even non-profit organisations. By harnessing the collective expertise and resources of these diverse stakeholders, we can formulate more comprehensive and effective health strategies. Collaborative efforts can drive innovation, pooling resources and knowledge to tackle public health challenges more efficiently.

Moreover, AI-driven population health analytics can contribute significantly to policy-making. Policymakers can rely on AI-generated insights to design evidence-based health policies. Whether it's formulating vaccination strategies, planning for healthcare infrastructure, or allocating budgets, data-driven decisions are likely to be more effective and equitable. The ability to back policy choices with hard data can also enhance public trust in health initiatives—an essential component for successful implementation.

In conclusion, population health analytics powered by AI is an evolving field with enormous potential. We're standing at the brink of a health revolution, driven by data and technology. While challenges exist, they can be met with careful planning, ethical considerations, and a commitment to continuous learning. As AI analytics becomes more refined, we can expect to see a profound impact on how public health is managed globally, ushering in an era of smarter, more proactive health interventions that benefit all of society.

Chapter 10:
AI in Clinical Specialities

Just when you think AI has dazzled us enough, it dives deeper into clinical specialities, sprucing up radiology with algorithms that can pinpoint anomalies in imaging scans quicker than you can say "MRI". In the realm of precision medicine, AI's prowess shines brightly, customising treatment plans down to the molecular level and making a mockery of one-size-fits-all approaches. Then, there's mental health—a field so nuanced that even the most skilled therapists sometimes struggle. Here, AI steps in with predictive models and virtual assistants that provide immediate support and flag potential crises before they escalate. While this might make it sound like we're outsourcing empathy to machines, it's really about augmenting human capability, letting clinicians focus on aspects that machines can't touch—at least, not yet.

AI Applications in Radiology

Walk into any modern radiology department today, and you might just feel you're stepping into the future. You see, radiology, the backbone for so much of medical diagnostics, is undergoing quite the renaissance thanks to artificial intelligence (AI). Lurking behind those mammoth imaging machines are algorithms working tirelessly to push boundaries and uncover what the human eye might miss. But is it all sunshine and rainbows?

Well, consider this: radiologists spend hours pouring over intricate images, meticulously looking for the slightest hint of abnormality. Enter AI. Armed with machine learning and deep-learning algorithms, it's almost as if these digital Sherlocks have a magnifying glass that can zoom in on nuances, much faster and often more accurately than their human counterparts. These algorithms are trained on millions of images, enabling them to recognize various diseases, from a simple fracture to more insidious cancers. What's more, some can even suggest a prognosis based on historical data. Impressive, right?

Yet, you'll find the implementation of AI in radiology isn't about replacing the venerable radiologist. Instead, it's more akin to having a hyper-competent assistant who isn't limited by human fatigue or cognitive biases. Radiologists now have AI-powered tools to sift through volumes of images quickly, flagging areas that require closer examination. This doesn't just augment their efficiency; it also enhances diagnostic accuracy, leading to better patient outcomes. Curiously, with AI's ability to identify subtler anomalies, early detection sees a significant boost—a stitch in time, some might say.

On a closer look, AI's applications in radiology extend beyond image interpretation. Consider the intricate and time-consuming task of registering images, aligning them so that snapshots taken at different times can be compared effectively. AI algorithms are making this process significantly faster and more accurate, which is no small feat given the complexities of human anatomy and the potential for slight movements between scans. Imagine what radiologists can achieve when freed from such painstaking tasks.

Alright, let's touch upon a few breeds of AI making waves in the radiology realm. First up, we have convolutional neural networks (CNNs). These are particularly adept at image analysis and have proven their mettle in detecting conditions like pneumonia on chest X-rays or identifying brain tumours on MRIs. Next, there's natural language processing (NLP), which sifts through electronic health records and radiology reports to extract pertinent clinical information that could add context to imaging findings. It's like having a library assistant with a photographic memory. Then there's the role of AI in predictive analytics, offering probabilistic assessments of disease progression, which is increasingly invaluable for chronic condition management.

That's not to say there aren't hurdles to overcome. The road to full-scale AI integration is fraught with regulatory challenges, interoperability issues, and a steep learning curve for medical professionals. Data privacy remains a constant concern, as does the need for transparency in AI decision-making processes. Radiologists are wary of "black box" algorithms, where the decision-making pathway is as clear as mud. For AI to gain widespread acceptance, its suggestions need to be interpretable, making sure the human remains the final arbiter in diagnostic decisions.

Now, before we get carried away by the techno-utopian narrative, let's not forget the human aspects at play. Radiologists aren't just passive recipients of AI's wisdom. Ongoing training is essential to help them understand and effectively use AI tools. Consequently, medical schools are increasingly including AI training in their curriculums. This symbiotic relationship between man and machine is essential to reap the full benefits AI promises.

Whilst AI can process and analyse data at a breakneck speed, its ability to understand the nuances of patient care and the ethical levels of decision-making is still very much a work in progress. Take, for example, incidental findings—those unexpected anomalies that fall outside the primary focus of the exam. A radiologist's experience and intuition often play a major role in deciding the significance of these blips on the radar. Can AI replicate this level of discernment? As it stands, that's questionable.

Geopolitics adds yet another layer to this complex mosaic. Like it or not, access to this cutting-edge AI technology is uneven across the globe. While some developed nations are eager adopters, resource constraints and infrastructural challenges mean that less affluent regions lag. The risk here is a widening healthcare disparity, something that policymakers and global health organisations must tackle head-on.

Despite these challenges, it's difficult to be anything but optimistic about the future of AI in radiology. The potential for reducing diagnostic errors, enhancing early detection, and improving patient outcomes presents a compelling case for its adoption. Imagine a future where AI not only complements radiologists but also collaborates seamlessly with other specialities, integrating various data points to create a holistic view of a patient's health. We're talking about a brave new world of precision medicine, where the margin for error dramatically shrinks, and tailored treatment protocols become the norm rather than the exception.

To sum up, AI in radiology is not just a tech upgrade; it's a paradigm shift. It's as much about augmenting human capabilities as it is about heralding a new era in medical diagnostics. And while the journey is filled with obstacles and ethical quandaries, the destination promises nothing short of a revolution. Radiology, it seems, is on the cusp of its most transformative phase yet, with AI as its trusty compadre. Now, isn't that something to anticipate?

AI-Assisted Precision Medicine

Precision medicine, a game-changer in the healthcare sector, is reaching unprecedented heights with AI assistance. By integrating big data, genomics, and advanced algorithms, AI is not just pushing boundaries; it is redefining them. The confluence of these technologies paves the way for bespoke treatment plans tailored to the genetic makeup of individual patients, thereby enhancing the efficacy of medical interventions.

Central to AI-assisted precision medicine is the ability to delve into genetic profiles at a granular level. Through machine learning algorithms, vast amounts of genomic data can be analysed swiftly, identifying mutations and predicting susceptibility to specific diseases. This isn't just theory. It's already being utilised in cancer treatments where AI can distinguish between tumour types, predict their progression, and suggest personalised therapies. These advancements don't merely save time; they can save lives.

Imagine having a healthcare system where treatments are not just reactive but proactive. Early detection is one of the crowning achievements of AI in this field. By employing intricate algorithms, AI systems can pinpoint anomalies in genetic sequences long before symptoms even surface. Predictive analytics can flag potential health risks based on genetic predispositions, allowing for early interventions that could dramatically improve patient outcomes. This precision-driven approach marks a sharp departure from traditional, more generalised medical treatments.

Personalisation doesn't stop at the genetic level. AI also leverages a multitude of other data points—from lifestyle factors to environmental exposures—to create a comprehensive health profile for each patient. The ability to process and integrate these diverse data sets ensures that recommendations are not just based on genetics but consider the individual holistically. This multidimensional analysis leads to treatment plans that are as unique as the patients themselves.

Of course, the utility of AI in precision medicine goes beyond diagnostics and treatment recommendations. It also makes drug development more precise. Pharmaceutical companies are leveraging AI to identify potential drug candidates and predict their efficacy and safety profiles rapidly. This accelerates the timeline from research to market, bringing life-saving drugs to patients faster than ever before.

One of the more compelling aspects is the democratisation of expertise. Not every healthcare facility has access to top-tier geneticists or oncologists. AI bridges this gap by making high-level insights available through user-friendly platforms. Thus, even remote clinics can offer advanced care that was previously confined to specialised institutions. This levelling of the playing field contributes to more equitable healthcare delivery.

Integration with electronic health records (EHR) is another area where AI shines. EHR systems, traditionally seen as cumbersome, are being revitalised through the infusion of AI technologies. Patterns and correlations that might elude human eyes are easily uncovered by AI, offering deeper insights into patient histories. With every scan, test, and click, the AI systems continue to learn, becoming more adept at providing spot-on recommendations.

However, it's not all smooth sailing. Ethical considerations loom large in the realm of AI-assisted precision medicine. Data privacy is a significant concern, given the sensitive nature of genetic information. There's also the question of accuracy and the potential for algorithmic bias. If the training data is flawed, the AI outputs will be, too. Hence, continuous validation and rigorous scrutiny of AI models are imperative to maintain trust and reliability.

The role of healthcare professionals is evolving in this AI-enhanced landscape. Doctors and nurses are transitioning from being sole decision-makers to becoming interpreters of the insights generated by AI systems. This collaborative model aims to combine human intuition with machine precision. Continuous education and training are essential to equip medical professionals with the skills needed to navigate this new era of healthcare.

Amidst all the technological wizardry, one must not overlook the patient's role. Engaging patients in their healthcare journey has never been more critical. With the help of AI, patients gain greater access to information about their conditions and treatment options. This transparency fosters a sense of empowerment and encourages adherence to personalised treatment plans. Patient portals driven by AI can provide real-time updates and recommendations, putting control directly into the hands of individuals.

AI-assisted precision medicine has the potential to redefine healthcare as we know it. By integrating genetic data with advanced analytics, predictive modelling, and personalised care, it promises a future where medical interventions are more accurate, effective, and equitable. While challenges such as data privacy and algorithmic bias need to be meticulously managed, the benefits of this technology are immense. As we continue to push the envelope on what's possible, the dream of a healthcare system tailored to the individual, capable of preemptively addressing health concerns, is becoming our new reality.

AI in mental Health

Artificial Intelligence isn't just transforming the physical aspects of healthcare; it's increasingly becoming a crucial player in the realm of mental health as well. In a society where mental well-being is just as vital as physical health, AI's potential to revolutionise mental health care is monumental. From chatbots providing instant cognitive behavioural therapy (CBT) to machine learning algorithms capable of predicting mental health crises, the integration of AI in mental health is advancing rapidly.

The struggles surrounding mental health are widespread and deeply personal, affecting millions each year. Traditional mental health care is often fraught with barriers, including stigma, a lack of accessible services, and the subjective nature of mental health diagnoses. AI seeks to address some of these chronic issues by offering scalable, personalised, and data-driven solutions.

One of the most exciting developments is the use of AI-driven chatbots that can engage users in therapeutic conversations. These chatbots are designed to mimic human emotions and can offer initial support and coping strategies for those struggling with anxiety, depression, or any number of mental health issues. They provide an accessible entry point for people who might be hesitant to seek traditional therapy. Crucially, these virtual therapists are available 24/7, offering instant support when it's most needed.

For instance, platforms like Woebot use natural language processing to engage in CBT, aiming to shift negative thought patterns. Users get immediate responses and customised advice, making mental health support more immediate and personalised than ever before. Unlike a human therapist, these AI systems can handle multiple users simultaneously, broadening the reach of mental health services exponentially.

However, chatbots are only the tip of the iceberg. AI is also making strides in more profound and predictive aspects of mental health. Algorithms analysing social media activity, sleep patterns, and even smartphone usage can identify behavioural anomalies indicative of mental health issues. For example, machine learning models can detect language patterns symptomatic of depression or suicidal ideation.

These predictive capabilities have enormous implications for preventative care. Imagine a scenario where a combination of mobile app data points triggers an alert to a healthcare provider, recommending a check-in with the patient. Such early interventions could be life-changing, or even life-saving, preventing a downward spiral before it becomes critical.

Moreover, these technologies aren't just hypothetical. Real-world applications are already demonstrating their efficacy. For instance, researchers at various institutions are exploring how AI can identify symptoms of post-traumatic stress disorder (PTSD) through voice analysis. By picking up on subtle stress markers in speech, the technology aims to assist clinicians in making faster, more accurate diagnoses.

Professional settings are also benefiting from AI's capabilities. Telemedicine platforms using AI can sort through patient symptoms to provide doctors with a more accurate picture of a client's mental health status. This assists clinicians in creating precise and timely treatment plans, reducing the subjective element that often bogs down mental health diagnosis and treatment.

AI's integration into mental health care does come with its challenges. Issues around data privacy and the ethical use of AI persist, echoing broader concerns within the digital age. Ensuring the confidentiality and security of sensitive mental health information is paramount. Additionally, there's the risk of over-reliance on technology, potentially reducing the human touch that is often indispensable in therapeutic relationships.

Despite these challenges, the role of AI in mental health is expected to grow. Policies ensuring ethical guidelines and proper use will need to evolve alongside these technologies. Researchers and clinicians will also need to stay up-to-date with ongoing advancements, with training programs integrating new AI tools and methods into standard practices.

Looking ahead, the fusion of AI with wearable technology and neuroimaging could offer even more detailed insights into mental health. Devices that monitor physiological indicators like heart rate variability or cortisol levels could provide real-time data, helping in the early detection of stress or anxiety disorders. Imagining a future where your smartwatch could alert you to an impending mood shift isn't far-fetched—it's on the horizon.

In essence, the advent of AI in mental health brings renewed hope and possibilities. From expanding access to mental health care to providing more accurate and personalised treatments, the potential benefits are substantial. While challenges remain, the transformative impact of AI on mental health services is a significant step towards a more compassionate and effective healthcare system.

AI in Human Reproduction

AI's ingress into human reproduction isn't just impending; it's already transforming the landscape. From assisting in diagnosing infertility causes to optimising in-vitro fertilisation (IVF) procedures, AI is poised to make significant strides. Think of it as a trained observer with millions of infertility cases at its disposal, discerning patterns too subtle for human doctors to catch. It's like having Sherlock Holmes as your fertility specialist.

One of the most profound applications of AI in human reproduction is enhancing the success rates of IVF. A procedure that's often emotionally and financially taxing, IVF has a success rate that can vary for myriad reasons—many of which aren't apparent at first glance. AI models can analyse vast datasets from previous cycles to predict the likelihood of success for future cycles, essentially tailoring the process to the nuances of individual patients. By scrutinising the embryo quality, genetic information, and even patient health records, AI can propose the most viable embryos for transfer. This is nothing short of revolutionary.

Then there's the matter of sperm analysis. Traditionally, this has been evaluated by embryologists, who perform a visual assessment under a microscope. While effective, this method is inevitably subject to human error and variability. Enter AI algorithms, which can assess sperm morphology and motility with remarkable precision. These systems can process and learn from thousands of sperm samples, yielding analytics that far surpass human capabilities.

Additionally, AI can offer invaluable support in diagnosing conditions leading to infertility. Machine learning algorithms can analyse a patient's medical history, hormone levels, and even lifestyle factors to flag issues that may be the root cause. Conditions like polycystic ovarian syndrome (PCOS) and endometriosis, for instance, can be better understood and managed through AI's pattern recognition capabilities.

Automated counselling might sound like a stretch, but AI-driven virtual assistants are already providing mental support to patients undergoing fertility treatments. These tools can offer 24/7 support, addressing concerns and questions that otherwise would require timely human intervention. A bit of AI-guided empathy can go a long way, arguably more consistent than the erratic schedules of human counsellors.

A burgeoning frontier is AI's role in genetic screening. Preimplantation genetic testing (PGT) can identify chromosomal abnormalities before embryo implantation. The effectiveness and accuracy of PGT can be substantially augmented by AI algorithms, which can analyse genetic data more quickly and accurately than current methods allow.

But let's not race ahead without acknowledging the potential issues. Data privacy remains a concern. The idea that intimate health information could be stored and potentially mishandled is daunting. Then there's the ethical dilemma of how much intervention is too much—are we heading towards a future where AI makes decisions that edge us into the realm of "designer babies"? Heavy questions that demand careful contemplation.

Overall, AI's involvement in human reproduction is a scientific marvel that exemplifies its wide-reaching potential. The advances are rapid and the implications vast, suggesting a future where the heartbreak of infertility could be substantially mitigated, guided by the discerning eye of artificial intelligence. So, as we embark on this technological journey, it's crucial to balance innovation with ethical considerations, ensuring we tread this new path responsibly.

AI in the Field of Surgery is revolutionising the operating theatre in ways that were once the realm of science fiction. Today, we're witnessing an era where machines don't just assist surgeons—they actively alter the dynamics and outcomes of surgical procedures. This isn't about replacing skilled hands with a robot. Instead, it's an intricate dance where human expertise and machine precision harmonise to redefine healthcare standards.

The advent of robotic-assisted surgeries has already made waves. Robots, controlled by surgeons through a console, provide unparalleled precision, enabling minimally invasive surgeries with drastically reduced recovery times. Consider the Da Vinci Surgical System, which has garnered significant attention. It extends the range of human motion, allowing surgeons to perform complex tasks through tiny incisions with robotic arms that are steadier and more precise than any human hand could achieve.

Moreover, artificial intelligence is being used to enhance these robotic systems further. Machine learning algorithms analyse vast datasets to improve surgical techniques, predict potential complications, and recommend optimal surgical pathways. For instance, AI-driven analytics can scrutinise patient data and previous surgical outcomes to forecast which methods would yield the best results for specific individuals.

Beyond robotic assistance, there's the realm of pre-surgical planning where AI's influence is profound. Advanced imaging technologies integrate with AI to create 3D models of patient anatomy. Surgeons can rehearse complex operations in a virtual environment, visualising every step before making the first incision. This practice doesn't just bolster confidence but significantly enhances the precision and likelihood of a successful outcome.

AI's contribution to intraoperative guidance cannot be overstated either. Systems equipped with computer vision and augmented reality (AR) provide real-time support. For example, AR glasses can overlay critical information onto the surgeon's visual field, highlighting crucial anatomical structures and helping to avoid vital organs and blood vessels. The combination of AI and AR elevates the surgeon's situational awareness, making procedures safer and more efficient.

Post-surgery, AI continues to play a pivotal role. Predictive algorithms monitor recovery, flagging any signs of potential complications like infections or irregular vital signs. These systems ensure interventions are timely, mitigating risks before they escalate into serious issues. By providing a continuous stream of insights, AI ensures patients not only recover faster but also with fewer setbacks.

Despite these advancements, it's worth noting the nuances and challenges that accompany AI in surgery. Ethical considerations, such as decision-making autonomy and liability in case of errors, require thorough deliberation. Additionally, the integration of AI into surgical practice demands substantial training and adaptation from healthcare professionals. Building trust in a system where a machine plays a crucial role in human health is no small feat.

But the potential benefits far outweigh the hurdles. AI is poised to make surgeries safer, more precise, and less invasive. This transformative technology, while still evolving, offers a compelling glimpse into a future where surgical outcomes are more predictable and successful, ultimately saving lives and enhancing the quality of patient care.

Chapter 11:
Transforming the NHS

The Care Quality Commission (CQC), the regulatory body ensuring healthcare standards across England, is on the cusp of transformation with the advent of artificial intelligence. Imagine this: AI stepping into the arena, meticulously analysing vast amounts of data to provide real-time, unbiased assessments of hospital and clinic performances. The leverage of predictive analytics, for example, could not only detect patterns of non-compliance early but also forecast potential areas of concern before they materialise into serious issues.

Consider the monumental task of inspecting and assessing countless healthcare facilities. With AI's capability to crunch through enormous datasets and flag areas needing immediate attention, inspectors' workloads would significantly lighten. Consequently, the focus can shift from merely ticking boxes to genuinely enhancing patient care and safety. Algorithms that learn from historical data can propose tailor-made improvement plans, fitting each facility's unique challenges and needs.

Yet, this transformation isn't just about efficiency—it's also about fairness and consistency. Humans, whether we like it or not, can be swayed by biases, fatigue, or even the weather. AI offers a level of impartiality that's hard to achieve otherwise. Each inspection, each assessment can be held to uniform standards, eliminating variations that sometimes undermine the credibility of regulation.

Of course, blending AI with the CQC's traditional practices won't be without its challenges. Trust in the system, transparency in AI decision-making, and data security concerns will need to be scrupulously addressed. Training the workforce to effectively collaborate with AI tools and integrating new technologies smoothly into existing frameworks are vital steps. But the potential rewards—a more responsive, fair, and proactive regulatory system—promise to drive the NHS into a future where patient care continuously evolves to new heights of excellence.

Specific Applications within the NHS

The journey of integrating AI into the NHS is both riveting and daunting, with myriad applications poised to transform the landscape of healthcare delivery. AI isn't just about pretentious concepts and far-off dreams; it's about tangible, everyday improvements that can save lives, cut costs, and make the healthcare experience more humane and efficient.

Let's start with diagnostics, an area where AI promises to be a game-changer. AI can scan through medical imaging far more quickly and accurately than a human could. Take the case of radiology. Machine learning algorithms can sift through millions of X-rays, CT scans, and MRIs, identifying anomalies that could be easily overlooked by the human eye. In hospitals across the NHS, pilot projects are already demonstrating impressive results. Dr. Clare Marx, a noted radiologist, remarked, "AI is like having an extra pair of expert eyes that never tire."

Moving on to predictive analytics, this is another arena where the NHS stands to benefit substantially. By crunching vast amounts of patient data, AI can predict who might develop chronic diseases such as diabetes or cardiovascular conditions. This kind of insight allows for early intervention, which is not only cost-effective but also improves the patient's quality of life significantly. Imagine a scenario where your GP informs you that you're at risk of developing Type 2 diabetes, well before any symptoms manifest. Early warnings can lead to lifestyle changes and preventative measures, reducing the strain on NHS resources in the long run.

Then there's personalised medicine, tailored to a patient's unique genetic makeup. It sounds like sci-fi, but it's not far off from becoming mainstream within the NHS. AI algorithms can analyse your genetic data to recommend specific treatments that are more likely to work for you. An example can be seen in oncology, where tailored treatment plans can significantly improve patient outcomes. This is real, actionable science, not just wishful thinking.

Administrative efficiencies may not sound as exciting as cutting-edge medical treatments, but they are crucial for a mammoth organisation like the NHS. AI can streamline administrative tasks, freeing up healthcare professionals to focus on what they do best: caring for patients. Natural language processing (NLP) tools can handle patient intake forms, schedule appointments, and even manage billing. The result? A smoother, faster experience for both patients and staff. Professor Nigel Scott, a healthcare management expert, noted, "The real beauty of AI in administration is its ability to cut through red tape and reduce bottlenecks." For an overstretched public health system, these improvements can make a world of difference.

Touching upon patient engagement, AI-driven virtual health assistants, like chatbots, offer round-the-clock help. These bots can provide basic medical advice, remind patients to take their medication, or answer questions about symptoms, freeing up GPs and nurses to tackle more complex cases. According to a study published by the BMJ, the implementation of AI chatbots in primary care settings led to a 20% reduction in patient wait times.

Another exciting application within the NHS is the use of wearable technology for remote patient monitoring. Devices such as smartwatches and fitness trackers can collect data on a patient's heart rate, activity levels, and even sleep patterns. This data can then be analysed by AI to detect early signs of potential health issues. What's remarkable is how these technologies empower patients to take an active role in their own health management, often catching problems before they require hospital admission.

Even in the operating theatre, AI is becoming an invaluable ally. Robotic surgery systems, guided by AI, are already assisting surgeons in performing precise and minimally invasive procedures. These robots aren't the stuff of dystopian nightmares but are instead practical tools that ensure higher accuracy and faster recovery times. Surgeons at the Royal Free Hospital in London have successfully used AI-assisted robotic systems in complex surgeries, reducing operating times and improving patient outcomes.

And let's not overlook mental health services, where AI can offer some unexpected but critical support. For instance, AI algorithms can help flag patients who might be at risk of depression or anxiety based on their interactions with digital health platforms. These tools can also provide support via virtual counselling sessions, making mental health services more accessible, especially given the strain on traditional mental health services within the NHS. Dr. Robin Murray, a psychiatrist at the South London and Maudsley NHS Foundation Trust, said, "AI can extend the reach of our mental health services, providing timely interventions and helping to reduce social stigma."

Of course, implementing AI within the NHS isn't without its challenges. Data privacy remains a significant concern, as does the need for rigorous training and education for healthcare professionals. The legal and ethical considerations are also intricate, demanding a careful balance between innovation and patient safety. Yet, despite these hurdles, the potential benefits are too compelling to ignore.

The financial impact can't be understated either. The NHS faces constant funding pressures, and AI offers a way to do more with less. By optimizing resource allocation and reducing inefficiencies, AI has the potential to save the NHS billions annually. A report by the Institute of Global Health Innovation at Imperial College London estimated that AI could save the NHS up to £3 billion a year by improving prevention, diagnostics, and operational efficiencies. Imagine what could be achieved if even a fraction of these savings were reinvested into patient care.

In summary, the specific applications of AI within the NHS are vast and varied, each offering unique benefits that address some of the most pressing challenges in healthcare today. From diagnostics and predictive analytics to personalised medicine and administrative efficiencies, AI holds the promise of a future where healthcare is more intelligent, more efficient, and more patient-centered. These aren't just theoretical applications; they are real, practical solutions already being tested and implemented within the NHS. If harnessed effectively, AI could truly revolutionize healthcare as we know it, making the future of the NHS one of innovation and improved patient outcomes.

Potential Benefits and Challenges

The NHS, Britain's proud and longstanding institution, is on the brink of transformation with the integration of AI technologies. The potential benefits of incorporating AI into the NHS are numerous and monumental. However, where there are opportunities, challenges are inevitably close behind, playing the part of the necessary adversary in this tale of progress.

Let's start with the benefits. AI has the potential to bring efficiencies that the NHS has hitherto only dreamed of. For one, diagnostic accuracy could see unprecedented improvements. Technologies like machine learning can scrutinise medical images with a level of detail that rivals, and in some cases outstrips, even the most seasoned radiologists. This can significantly reduce the rate of misdiagnosis, which is a persistent problem in medical practice.

Moreover, AI can facilitate more personalised treatment plans. By analysing vast amounts of genetic data, AI-powered systems can help identify the best therapeutic protocols for individual patients, thereby moving away from the "one-size-fits-all" approach that characterises much of current medical practice. Tailoring treatments in this way can lead to better patient outcomes and possibly even lower healthcare costs over time.

Ultimately, the way AI can optimise administrative tasks is nothing short of game-changing. From scheduling appointments to managing patient records, AI can take over routine, time-consuming tasks that often bog down healthcare professionals. This leaves more room for them to focus on what they do best: providing care.

However, as promising as these benefits sound, they come with a litany of challenges that cannot be ignored. The foremost challenge is the issue of data privacy. The NHS houses an unimaginable amount of personal data, and integrating AI systems necessitates the use of this data. Ensuring this data is kept secure and private is not just a logistical challenge but also a moral imperative. The road to AI integration is paved with sensitive information, and one misstep could result in catastrophic data breaches.

Another significant challenge lies in the ethical implications of AI decision-making. When an AI system recommends a particular treatment plan or makes a diagnosis, who is accountable if something goes wrong? The healthcare professional, the AI developer, or the NHS itself? These are ethical grey areas that require careful consideration and robust policy-making.

Training and education represent another sizeable hurdle. Healthcare professionals are, by and large, not trained in the intricacies of AI algorithms and machine learning models. Introducing AI into the NHS will necessitate comprehensive training programs to ensure that staff can effectively use these new tools. This is neither quick nor cheap and adds yet another layer of complexity to the already challenging integration process.

Resource allocation for such a large-scale transformation is also a sticking point. The NHS is famously strapped for cash, and the initial financial outlay required for AI integration could be steep. Not all trusts within the NHS may have the resources to adopt these new technologies simultaneously, leading to potential inequalities in the quality of care across different regions.

There's also the matter of public trust. The idea of a machine making decisions about one's health can be a hard pill to swallow. Gaining the trust of the public and healthcare professionals is crucial for the successful implementation of AI. Any error or flaw in the system can significantly erode this trust, making it a precarious balancing act.

Moreover, the NHS workforce may also view AI as a threat rather than an aid. There's an inherent fear that AI could replace human jobs, particularly in fields like diagnostic radiology and pathology. While AI is more about augmentation than replacement, these fears are not without merit and need to be addressed transparently.

Finally, the pace of technological advancements could itself pose a challenge. AI technologies evolve rapidly, often outpacing the policies and infrastructure designed to support them. Keeping up with such rapid advancements requires continuous updates to policies, standards, and training programs, further complicating the integration process.

In conclusion, the potential benefits of integrating AI into the NHS and Care Quality Commission, the Quality Regulators are vast and varied, holding the promise of revolutionising healthcare delivery. However, the path to realising these benefits is fraught with challenges that must be addressed meticulously. From data privacy and ethical considerations to training and resource allocation, the barriers are significant but not insurmountable. In navigating these challenges, the NHS must strive to balance innovation with caution, ensuring that the transformative power of AI benefits all without compromising the core values of this venerable institution.

Chapter 12:
The Future of AI in Global Healthcare

The future landscape of global healthcare is set to undergo transformative leaps thanks to AI, and it's high time we embrace this change with cautious optimism. Emerging trends and innovations, ranging from sophisticated diagnostic algorithms to autonomous surgical robots, promise to redefine how healthcare services are delivered worldwide. But it's not just about flashy tech—AI's long-term impact on global health could be monumental, especially in remote and underserved areas where medical professionals are scarce. With these advancements, healthcare can become more predictive, personalised, and efficient, ultimately bridging gaps in access and quality of care. While ethical and legal hurdles remain, the potential for AI-driven improvement in global health systems is undeniable. As we look ahead, the integration of AI in everyday medical practice isn't just inevitable; it's imperative for a healthier, more connected world.

Emerging Trends and Innovations

The landscape of global healthcare has been a fertile ground for innovations, particularly when it comes to the realm of artificial intelligence (AI). While we marvel at the technological advancements already making waves, it's crucial to keep an eye on what's coming next. AI, much like the proverbial iceberg, has a lot more lurking beneath the surface. So, let's delve into the emergent trends and innovations shaping the future of healthcare.

One of the most dazzling trends in AI healthcare is the development of **predictive algorithms** that can anticipate medical conditions before they manifest. These algorithms scrutinise a vast array of data, including genetic information, lifestyle choices, and environmental factors, to predict ailments ranging from diabetes to cardiovascular diseases. This shift towards preventive healthcare aims to diagnose and address problems before they necessitate serious medical intervention.

Blockchain technology, frequently associated with cryptocurrencies, is finding its way into healthcare, creating a new paradigm in data security. With patient data becoming increasingly a cyber-target, blockchain offers an immutable ledger for data exchange, making every transaction traceable and transparent. This not only enhances data security but also paves the way for extensive data sharing and interoperability across different healthcare systems globally.

Let's not ignore the strides being made in **robotic surgery**. Robots have been part of surgical rooms for decades, but recent advancements are pushing the boundaries of what's possible. AI-driven robots can now perform highly intricate surgeries with precision often unattainable by human hands. By minimising invasiveness and reducing recovery times, these robotic assistants could make surgeries safer and more efficient.

Another intriguing area is the use of **AI in mental health**. Algorithms can now analyse text or speech to assess the mental well-being of individuals. By monitoring subtle cues, AI can gauge stress levels, depression, and other mental health conditions, offering timely interventions. These advancements could be crucial in breaking down the stigma surrounding mental health by providing accessible, non-intrusive diagnostic tools.

Natural Language Processing (NLP) is also making waves. NLP algorithms are becoming more sophisticated, enabling better communication between machines and humans. This not only assists doctors in diagnosing conditions more accurately but also plays a vital role in patient interaction. Virtual health assistants equipped with NLP can provide personalised advice, schedule appointments, and even offer emotional support, making healthcare more holistic.

Wearable technology is another booming trend. With the integration of AI, wearables move beyond basic fitness trackers to become comprehensive health monitors. These devices can track a wide range of metrics, from heart rate variability to blood oxygen levels, transmitting this data to healthcare providers in real-time. This continuous flow of information allows for proactive healthcare management, turning reactive treatment into proactive wellness.

One area that can't be overlooked is the **integration of AI with genomics**. AI algorithms are being employed to decode the vast amount of data contained within the human genome. This decoding helps in identifying genetic markers for diseases, aiding in the creation of personalised treatment plans. Imagine a world where your medical care is tailored to your genetic makeup—this is no longer science fiction but an emerging reality.

The democratisation of medical knowledge through AI is another fascinating trend. Machine learning models are analysing a plethora of medical literature at speeds no human could manage, summarising key findings and ensuring that healthcare professionals are up-to-date with the latest research. This democratisation extends to patients as well, with AI applications offering insights that empower individuals to take control of their own health.

In terms of diagnostics, AI is championing the cause of *remote monitoring and consultations*. With advancements in telemedicine, AI-backed platforms can offer initial consultations, reducing the need for in-person visits. This is particularly beneficial in rural or underserved areas, where access to healthcare is often limited. These platforms are designed to identify urgent cases that require immediate physical intervention, ensuring that no patient is left behind.

Furthermore, **AI is revolutionising clinical trials**. The traditional model of clinical trials is cumbersome and time-consuming, often taking years to yield results. AI's ability to analyse vast datasets quickly means that potential candidates for clinical trials can be identified more efficiently, the results can be interpreted more rapidly, and the timeline for developing new treatments can be significantly reduced.

Emerging trends also point towards the involvement of **AI in drug discovery**. Traditionally, discovering new drugs is a long, expensive, and labor-intensive process. AI can sift through existing chemicals and compounds to identify potential candidates for new drugs, predict their efficacy, and even suggest modifications to improve their performance. This could drastically cut down the time and cost involved in bringing new drugs to the market.

Another noteworthy innovation is in the field of **virtual reality (VR) and augmented reality (AR)**. These technologies, driven by AI, are being adopted for both training and treating patients. For example, VR simulations offer medical students and professionals lifelike scenarios to practice procedures without the risk of causing harm. Meanwhile, AR can assist surgeons in real-time by overlaying critical information during operations, enhancing precision.

AI's role in enhancing *patient experiences* is also not to be underestimated. From simplifying administrative tasks like scheduling and billing to offering personalised health recommendations, AI is making healthcare more user-friendly. Virtual health assistants can handle myriad daily interactions, ensuring that the human staff is freed up to focus on more complex and sensitive tasks.

Voice-enabled AI technology is another emerging trend. Devices like *Amazon's Alexa* and *Google Home* are not just smart home assistants but are becoming integral parts of healthcare ecosystems. These devices can remind patients to take their medications, monitor vital signs, and even facilitate quick communication with healthcare providers. Voice AI offers a hands-free, efficient way for patients to manage their health, especially beneficial for the elderly and those with limited mobility.

We're also seeing exciting developments in **nanotechnology**. Nano-bots, guided by AI algorithms, could one day navigate through the human body to perform precise tasks like targeting cancer cells or repairing tissue at the cellular level. While still in the experimental stages, this integration of AI and nanotechnology holds tremendous promise for the future of medicine.

The rise of **AI ethics** in healthcare is an emerging trend that's too significant to ignore. As AI systems become more involved in decision-making processes, questions around ethics, bias, and accountability are coming to the forefront. The healthcare sector is grappling with how to ensure that AI algorithms are transparent, fair, and unbiased. Establishing ethical guidelines and standards is crucial for fostering trust and ensuring that AI innovations are used responsibly.

A final area worth mentioning is the merging of **AI with biopharmaceuticals**. AI is helping in creating advanced biopharmaceuticals, including bi-specific antibodies, gene therapies, and even personalised vaccines. These treatments are not only more effective but can be tailored to individual patients, opening new frontiers in personalised medicine.

Long-Term Impact on Global Health

The long-term ramifications of AI in global healthcare have the potential to be transformative, promising a future where health services are more efficient, effective, and equitable. The integration of AI technologies can significantly alter the landscape of global health, affecting everything from disease prevention to healthcare delivery methods. But what does this really mean for the future? Well, some good, some bad, and some bizarrely uncharted territories.

For starters, AI has the seductive promise of enhancing disease prevention on a global scale. By leveraging AI's predictive analytics, healthcare systems can identify potential outbreaks before they spiral out of control. Imagine a world where diseases like malaria and cholera can be anticipated and nipped in the bud, saving millions of lives and billions in healthcare costs. Now, isn't that a future to look forward to?

AI also contributes to personalised medicine, where treatments are tailored to the individual rather than the masses. Genetic information, lifestyle choices, and even environmental factors can be integrated to offer bespoke healthcare plans. This ensures that each patient receives the most effective treatment, sidestepping the trial-and-error approach that often characterises contemporary medicine.

Yet, with great power comes great responsibility—and a few headaches. While AI offers a wealth of opportunities, its implementation might exacerbate existing inequalities. Wealthy nations could leap miles ahead in healthcare advancements, leaving poorer countries in the digital dust. The digital divide is a pressing concern, and effective implementation will require extensive international collaboration and investment to ensure that no one is left behind.

Moreover, AI in healthcare can drastically change the role of medical professionals. Think of it: fewer routine tasks, more time for complex problem-solving and patient care. But this shift won't be without consequences. It might lead to job displacement and necessitate a significant overhaul of medical education. Healthcare professionals will have to continuously adapt, learning to work alongside evolving AI technologies.

Additionally, the impact of AI on healthcare costs cannot be ignored. Initially, the integration of AI systems might skew the budget, making everything seem more expensive. However, in the long-run, the efficiencies created by AI can cut down operational costs, reduce errors, and improve patient outcomes. Consequently, healthcare may become more affordable and accessible for a global population.

But let's spare a thought for our ethical dilemmas. AI-driven healthcare is riddled with questions surrounding data privacy, security, and decision-making accountability. For instance, who is to blame if an AI diagnosis goes wrong? The programmer? The healthcare provider? The machine itself? There will need to be robust frameworks and regulations to tackle these intricacies.

In terms of public health, AI can be a game-changer. Tracking disease patterns, predicting outbreak trends, and implementing preventive measures on a global scale are more feasible with AI tools at our disposal. Imagine an AI system connected to global health networks, flagging potential pandemics well before they spread across borders. Amazing, right?

However, with the widespread application of AI, the data amassed is immense. Handling this tsunami of information requires sophisticated algorithms and infrastructures. This is where countries with advanced technological frameworks will shine, potentially monopolising global health data and creating new dynamics of power and influence in international health policies.

The long-term social impact can't go unnoticed either. AI's integration into healthcare might change public perceptions of health management. We'll see a shift towards more predictive and preventive care models. The emphasis would change from 'curing' illnesses to 'preventing' them. This could lead to healthier populations but also might result in a society too heavily reliant on technology for health solutions.

Looking at it from another angle, AI has the power to democratise healthcare information. By providing patients with better, more accurate information, AI can lead to more informed health decisions. People will be empowered to take control of their health in ways previously unimaginable. More personalised health tools, like smartwatches and apps that monitor vital signs, can also play a pivotal role in chronic disease management, thereby reducing hospital readmissions and improving the quality of life.

On the molecular front, AI's role in genomics is getting a spotlight. Precision medicine becomes more attainable when AI can parse through genetic codes and predict potential health issues long before they manifest. This revolution in early diagnosis and customised treatment plans will herald a new age of preemptive healthcare.

All of this might sound like a futuristic utopia or a sci-fi movie but integrating AI in healthcare is more pragmatic and grounded than it seems. It's a slow, meticulous process involving a myriad of stakeholders, from governments to private sector players. Each step forward needs to be scrutinised for practicality, ethics, and cost-effectiveness.

So, the long-term impact of AI in global healthcare is akin to a double-edged sword. It promises groundbreaking improvements but also brings along a multitude of challenges that need addressing. As we edge closer to this inevitable future, staying informed and engaged will be imperative. Who knows, the next health revolution might just come from the circuits and codes of artificial intelligence.

Conclusion

The confluence of artificial intelligence and the healthcare sector is not merely a matter of technological enhancement. It is a revolutionary transformation that stands to redefine healthcare paradigms and patient care models on a global scale. The intricacies of AI driving these changes are complex, yet the promise they hold is monumental. If there is one belief that underpins the entire discussion of AI in healthcare, it is that the future is both exciting and challenging.

The journey through understanding how AI can reform healthcare has made it abundantly clear: this marriage of technology and medicine offers unprecedented opportunities. However, with each opportunity comes a twin challenge. For instance, improving diagnostic accuracy with machine learning does offer the potential to save lives, yet it simultaneously raises questions about the reliability of AI predictions versus human judgment. It is crucial to navigate these waters carefully, ensuring that technological solutions do not alienate the human touch that is so central to healthcare.

Personalised medicine represents one of the most promising frontiers where AI can shine. The ability to tailor treatments to the individual patient based on myriad data points, such as genetic profiles and historical health data, can transform outcomes significantly. While the allure of such personalised care is strong, it is also true that the intricacies involved in data privacy and ethical considerations must not be overlooked. The ethical quandaries posed by the deep personalisation of medical care are not mere footnotes but core concerns that should guide future policy and implementation strategies.

Operational efficiency in hospitals isn't just a managerial achievement but a fundamental component of ensuring improved patient care. From resource allocation to streamlining administrative tasks, AI's role in optimising hospital management is invaluable. Yet, the transition phase poses its own set of problems. Resistance to change is natural, especially within established systems, and the integration of AI-driven tools and processes will likely face its share of operational hiccups and resistance from professionals accustomed to traditional methods.

Patient engagement has underestimated potential when viewed through the lens of AI. Virtual health assistants, wearable technologies, and remote monitoring systems are more than just gadgets—they are key to empowering patients and making healthcare more accessible. While the rise of virtual consultations and health monitoring apps makes for compelling headlines, the actual shift in patient behaviour and system readiness to support such technologies on a mass scale demands careful orchestration.

Ethical and legal considerations are the bedrock upon which any AI healthcare initiative must stand. In a domain as critical and sensitive as healthcare, issues of data privacy, security, and accountability cannot be secondary. They must form the foundational layers of AI deployment. The task is daunting, but rigorous standards and transparent policies can help navigate these ethical minefields. Ensuring that AI not only adheres to these standards but excels in reinforcing them is imperative.

In the training and education of healthcare professionals, integrating AI into medical curriculums is no longer optional; it is a necessity. Continuous learning and adaptation highlight the need for a workforce that's not just familiar with AI tools but proficient in leveraging them for optimal patient care. The challenge here is twofold: updating curriculum content at medical schools and ensuring that practising professionals continue to receive education and training in the latest AI advancements.

The role of AI in public health goes beyond individual treatments to encompass broader population health management. Tracking and managing epidemics through AI analytics can bolster public health responses, making them faster and more accurate. However, translating this potential into real-world efficacy requires robust infrastructures and collaborative data-sharing frameworks. The global health community must work cohesively to harness AI's full potential in public health contexts.

In clinical specialities, AI's applications are varied and profound. From enhancing imaging accuracy in radiology to assisting in precision medicine, AI is making inroads into fields traditionally reliant on clinician expertise. The synergy between human expertise and AI tools could redefine specialities, ensuring more precise diagnostics and personalised treatments. Yet, this revolution also brings the responsibility of equipping specialists with the tools and knowledge to integrate AI effectively into their practice.

Specific applications within national health systems, such as the NHS, illuminate the potential benefits and challenges in transforming public healthcare. The NHS stands as a testbed for broad application of AI in healthcare. The lessons learned here about both successes and pitfalls have global implications. Integration within such large systems highlights both the scalability of AI solutions and the logistical and bureaucratic hurdles that can impede progress.

The future of AI in global healthcare teems with emerging trends and innovations. This journey has only just begun, and the road ahead is filled with possibilities that are as thrilling as they are unpredictable.

The long-term impact on global health promises a landscape where AI not only complements but also augments human capabilities, creating a holistic and efficient healthcare ecosystem. However, realising this potential will require ongoing commitment, proactive policy-making, and an unwavering focus on ethical integrity.

In closing, the intersection of AI and healthcare is a landscape of immense possibility mingled with equally significant responsibility. As we look forward, the imperative is clear: to embrace and integrate artificial intelligence in ways that enhance, rather than replace, the human touch in medicine. By doing so, we'll usher in an era of healthcare that's not only advanced but also profoundly humane.

Appendix A:
Appendix

This section serves as a repository of supplemental materials and additional resources referenced throughout the book. For those wishing to delve deeper into the topics discussed, the following lists will provide a wealth of further reading and tools.

Additional Readings

- **Books:**

  - *The AI Revolution in Medicine: Artificial Intelligence in Medical Imaging* by Eric Topol

  - *Deep Medicine: How Artificial Intelligence Can Make Healthcare Human Again* by Eric Topol

  - *Artificial Intelligence in Healthcare* by Adam Bohr and Kaveh Memarzadeh

- **Articles:**

  - "The Role of Artificial Intelligence in Healthcare: A Systematic Review" from the Journal of Medical Internet Research

  - "Machine Learning in Healthcare: Data Trails and Algorithms" from The Lancet Digital Health

  - "Predictive Analytics for Chronic Disease Management" from Health Informatics Journal

Key Organisations and Websites

- <u>World Health Organization (WHO)</u>

- <u>National Institutes of Health (NIH)</u>

- <u>National Health Service (NHS)</u>

- <u>Healthcare Information and Management Systems Society (HIMSS)</u>

Software and Tools

- **TensorFlow:** An open-source machine learning framework.

- **IBM Watson Health:** AI-driven health insights and analytics platform.

- **Google Health:** Initiatives and research focused on applying AI to healthcare.

The above resources are recommended for those who are looking to expand their understanding and continue their exploration of how artificial intelligence is poised to transform the healthcare sector.

Additional Resources

Alright, so you've gone through the pool of information about AI's impending takeover of healthcare. If you're wondering where to dive deeper, the "Additional Resources" section is your golden ticket. We've rounded up a mix of articles, books, and websites that'll keep you well-informed and maybe even a little ahead of the curve.

- **Scientific Journals:** Don't miss out on seminal papers from journals like the *Journal of Artificial Intelligence Research* and *The Lancet Digital Health*. These publications frequently feature cutting-edge research about AI innovations in healthcare.

- **Academic Courses:** Institutions like Imperial College London and the University of Oxford offer online courses about AI applications in healthcare. These courses are perfect for gaining official credentials without quitting your day job.

- **Websites and Blogs:** Reputable websites like *AI in Healthcare* and blogs such as *Healthcare IT News* regularly publish articles that delve into the latest trends and breakthroughs. Bookmark these for your daily dose of AI in healthcare news.

- **Books:** To understand the broader implications and history of AI, consider reading books like *Artificial Intelligence: A Guide for Thinking Humans* by Melanie Mitchell and *Deep Medicine: How Artificial Intelligence Can Make Healthcare Human Again* by Eric Topol.

- **Podcasts and Webinars:** For those who prefer listening, there are podcasts such as *The AI Alignment* and *Future of Health*. Webinars hosted by healthcare conferences are also a valuable resource for learning from experts in the field.

- **Government and Organisation Reports:** Reports from NHS Digital and the World Health Organization offer insightful data and predictions about the integration of AI in healthcare systems worldwide.

Whether you're a healthcare professional, a tech enthusiast, or just someone curious about the future, these resources should help you stay informed and perhaps even inspired. Dive in and take advantage of everything available out there. Knowledge, after all, is power.

Glossary of Terms

The healthcare sector is rapidly evolving, and with the advent of technology, particularly Artificial Intelligence (AI), there are numerous new terms and concepts to get acquainted with. This glossary aims to provide definitions and descriptions for a range of terms that are pivotal in understanding the changes happening within the industry.

Artificial Intelligence (AI)

This refers to the simulation of human intelligence in machines designed to think and act like humans. In healthcare, AI can assist in diagnosing diseases, personalising treatment plans, and optimising hospital operations, among other things.

Machine Learning (ML)

A subset of AI, machine learning involves the use of algorithms and statistical models to enable systems to improve their performance on a task through experience. In healthcare, ML is often used for predictive analytics and disease diagnosis.

Genomics

The branch of molecular biology concerned with the structure, function, evolution, and mapping of genomes. AI-driven genomics aims to tailor medical treatments to individual genetic profiles.

Predictive Analytics

This involves using historical data, statistical algorithms, and machine learning techniques to predict future outcomes. In healthcare, predictive analytics can be used for early disease detection and personalised treatment plans.

Virtual Health Assistants

These are AI-powered tools that provide users with health-related information and services, usually through chatbots or virtual consultations. They aim to enhance patient engagement and make healthcare more accessible.

Wearable Technology

Devices that can be worn on the body to monitor health metrics such as heart rate, blood pressure, and activity levels. These devices can feed data into AI systems for real-time health monitoring and management.

Data Privacy and Security

Refers to the handling, processing, and protection of personal health information in compliance with regulations like GDPR. Ensuring data privacy and security is a major ethical consideration in the deployment of AI in healthcare.

Population Health Analytics

Involves the use of data analytics to improve health outcomes for groups of individuals. By analysing data on how certain conditions affect different populations, AI can help in managing epidemics and improving public health strategies.

Precision Medicine

A medical model that proposes the customisation of healthcare, with decisions and treatments tailored to the individual patient by integrating clinical and molecular data. AI plays a significant role in advancing precision medicine.

Continuous Learning

An on-going process where healthcare professionals keep updating their knowledge and skills. Integrating AI into medical curriculums is vital for preparing professionals to effectively use new technologies.

NHS (National Health Service)

The publicly funded healthcare system in the United Kingdom. AI applications within the NHS aim to enhance efficiency, patient care, and resource management.

Epidemic Tracking

The process of monitoring and analysing data related to the spread of infectious diseases. AI can significantly improve the accuracy and speed of epidemic tracking and response.

www.ingramcontent.com/pod-product-compliance
Lightning Source LLC
Chambersburg PA
CBHW051420280526
45785CB00003B/1102